Praise for
Garments of an Angel

Prepare to embark on an adventure where triumph
reigns over suffering... Thank you, Mrs. Hayes, for
being so open and honest...admonishing us to
never despise the journey!

Rev. Vivian Radden Moore, Ph.D.
Author, *Excellence is the Only Option*
Chesterfield, MO

Inspirational, the story shows how struggle and sacrifice
are rewarded. A *must read* for young women as they
begin their journey, and a *must read* for women
who are nearing the end of their journey.

Rev. Dovie Baumgardner
CEO, Women Sharing Wisdom Ministry
Cleveland, OH

It was difficult to put this book down and retire for the
evening while wondering what happened next. Mrs. Hayes
became transparent, revealing her emotions during those
times that were most difficult. Yet with a determination
to rise above her circumstances and see God, she
encourages her readers to do the same!

Rev. Dennis D. Cornelous
Associate Pastor, South Suburban Church of God
Homewood, IL

GARMENTS
OF AN ANGEL

By Rose Hayes

A My Heart Yours Publication

Publisher's Cataloging-in-Publication
(Provided by Quality Books, Inc.)

Hayes, Rose.
    Garments of an angel / by Rose Hayes.
    p. cm.
    LCCN 2004110140
    ISBN 1932721630

1. Hayes, Rose.
2. Christian biography--Illinois--Chicago.
3. African American women--Illinois--Chicago--Biography.
4. Chicago (Ill.)--Biography.   I. Title.

BR1725.H247A3 2004   277.73'11
                      QBI04-200474

SAN 256-0968

Forward

Everyone has a story. And in every story, there is a blessing for someone. For this reason I am sharing some of my most personal life experiences.

The wonderful love of all my children, grandchildren, and goddaughters, my friend Dottie and faithful Pastor Robbie, not to mention the healing balm I received from knowing Peter, enabled me to finish this writing I started many, many years ago.

I did not understand fully what Peter meant when he said, "It is not up to you, Renee. It is not up to you." Something happened to me that day, and today I understand.

I can now say each day, "Good morning, Holy Spirit. Thank You for speaking to my heart, for sending many angel encounters and *now the peace of God that surpasses all understanding shall keep my heart and mind." (Philippians 4:7)*

My God, my Father, You know my comings and goings. *The Lord shall preserve thy going out and thy coming in from this time forth, and even for evermore. (Psalm 121:8)*

My life is an open book. To You be the Glory!

Dedication

I dedicate this writing to:

My children,

Edward, Beverly (who preceded me in death),

Bettina, Gerald, and Eric

My godchildren,

Celestine and Albertha

And to *all* my beautiful grandchildren,

present and those to come

In His Time

In His time, in His time
He makes all things beautiful in His time
Lord, please show me every day
As You're teaching me Your way
That you do just what You say
In Your time

In Your time, in Your time
You make all things beautiful in Your time
Lord, my life to You I bring
May each song I have to sing
Be to You a lovely thing
In Your time

Diane Ball

*Your merciful love is higher than the heavens,
and Your truth reaches to the skies.*

Psalm 108:4

Prologue

My son Gamal, who worked at Stroger Hospital as an orthopedic technician, was one day called to the Operating Room to settle a dispute between an orthopedic student and another employee. He was needed as the union representative, and two nurses were asked to be present as witnesses.

Once the matter was settled, Gamal told the two nurses, "Listen, ladies, my mom is writing a book. You might be interested in purchasing a copy." One of the women asked, "What's the book about?" "It's mostly about angels in her life and also about land once owned by her father's foreparents," Gamal replied.

Where is the land?" this young lady asked. "In Dancy, Alabama," my son explained. "It's called the "Dancy Place." Laura, the other lady, now spoke up: "You and I might be related."

Gamal looked at her nametag, which read "Dancy." Then Laura gave Gamal a shock when she asked, "Did your Mom get money from the sawmill? My husband and son did."

"When was this?" Gamal asked. He knew about the will of Edwin Dancy, since he had heard his grandfather—my father—speak of it many times.

"The case went to court about twelve years ago, and was settled five years ago."

"I am sure my Mom would like to talk to you. Do you care if I give her your number?"

"You may give her my number. I would love to talk to her."

So several days later I had a long and very amiable conversation with Laura. She wanted to know if any of my family were musically inclined, since music was a Dancy trait. I told her of my great love for music, and how at times music transcends me into another world. I let her know that many of us had great voices.

There were so many things I wanted to ask Laura, especially about her husband's parents and grandparents: who were they? Where did they live? And when did they come to Chicago?

However, I did not feel comfortable asking her these questions or about the family inheritance. I knew that her in-laws, the Dancys, might not want her talking to me, since they were also writing a book and would most likely not want her sharing information that they were going to use, because my book would be published before theirs. When I called, Laura agreed to see me soon. However, even though I called several times and left messages, I did not get a response.

Still, I believe it was in God's plan for Gamal to be there on that day. It was mind-boggling to think that now, eight years after my dad's death, my son Gamal would come in contact with a Dancy this way. To think that 40 years ago, my dad's efforts to make known that he was a descendant of Edwin Dancy were not acknowledged.

Chapter 1

There was a time when my great-great-grandfather did not show up on the census, but by 1860, there he was: Edwin C. Dancy, age 49, a White farmer. The census reveals that Dancy owned real estate valued at $13,300 and a personal estate valued at $45,500. His birthplace—North Carolina—was also listed. Although he farmed, he was for some reason known as "*Dr.* Dancy."

No family was shown in the census listing. However, for a time, Dancy was married to Sabre, a Black Creek Indian who became my father's great-grandmother. However, there is no one alive who can tell us the exact dates of their marriage.

Dr. Dancy had five brothers: Henry, Lorenzo, Dallas, Nick, and Preston. After his wife Sabre's death, Dr. Dancy married again and was later listed as having two children: a daughter, Sallie, and a son, also named Preston. This Preston was father to Annie, and Annie was my father's mother.

Preston had a brother named Dallas, a son named Dallas, and a grandson (my father) named Dallas. The 1880 census of Pickens County, Alabama shows Preston Dancy: 38 years old, one son (Dallas), and five daughters.

Preston's daughter, Annie, eventually married Allen Jackson, and in the year 1911, my father was born to them. He was number 16 of 17 births. My grandfather Allen, an educated man, had a penmanship so perfect it looked like fine art, even though as far back as I can remember, he was blind.

ᴄᴦ

The town of Dancy, Alabama was named after Dr. Dancy, who died in July of 1891. The property then descended to his two children. When his son Preston died, he left numerous and unknown heirs.

In the late 1950s, my dad (Dallas) and two of his brothers learned that a large oil company was interested in "The Dancy Place"—land once owned by their foreparents. Since that land once belonged to Edwin Dancy's children, Sallie and Preston (my father's grandfather), my father believed that he and his brothers also held a claim to the land.

My dad and his brothers wrote to seven different judges in Alabama and to Governor George Wallace, trying to establish their connection to the family. In 1963, my Uncle Ed received letters from the National Archives and Records Service and the Assistant Attorney General. In 1965 my dad received a response from Governor Wallace, which read, in part:

> I […] regret that I cannot be of assistance to you. Unfortunately, the duties of my office are so numerous that I would not have time to investigate this matter personally and because of pressing duties, my staff is also unable to help you with this matter. I suggest that you retain an attorney to investigate this matter and then advise you concerning your best course of action.

Frustrated, the brothers wrote to the NAACP, who told them that someone had discovered that the brothers were Black. After that, no one would give out any information.

In all of this, the highlight for my dad was finally receiving a manila envelope from the White House from the office of Robert Kennedy. I do not know what Daddy did with that page. I remember reading it, because he was always showing it around. I do know that it talked about Sabre, which is how I know that she was from the Tribe of Black Creek Indians.

My father could not prove his relationship to the family, because he did not have a copy of his birth certificate. When he wrote the state of Alabama to request a copy, they refused, telling him the courthouse, along with its records, had burned down. His brother Edward met the same fate when he requested a copy of his birth certificate. A year later, however, another brother wrote and the state sent him a copy of his birth certificate. It seems to me that the courthouse was not burned down. That was just the excuse that most of the brothers received.

I would often appease my dad by letting him tell me over and over about his struggle for recognition as the great-grandson of Dr. Edwin Dancy. I listened, because he wanted to talk about his struggle. But my father did not get further because he did not have the funds to pursue his dream, and he said he and his brothers were afraid to go to Dancy, Alabama.

My father talked about this struggle many times. Often we would listen just out of respect. Dad wanted me to take up his fight. It made him happy to think I would do so. But it took all my energy to deal with the everyday problems of the twentieth century.

❧

All the letters and papers were precious to dad. He gave them to me and told me to take good care of them, because they were family history.

This book will be a legacy to my children. It will fulfill my Dad's wish that they know their roots and who their great-grandfather was.

Chicago Illinois
2/6/61

to whom it may concern I Dallas Jackson
was inform that My Grond father and 4 of his
Brothers was hiers to the Darcy Place noun
as Darcy alaboma the 5 Brothers was nome

1 Preston   Darcy
2 Henry   Darcy
3 lo Renza   Darcy
4 Dallas   Darcy
5 Nick   Darcy

My Grond father was Preston Darcy
My mother was Preston Darcy Doughter and
Preston Darcy had a Brother nome Dallas
                    a son + Dallas
          I am Grondson Dallas

Dallas Jackson
5422 So Prairie ave
Chicago 37 ill

Honable George Wallas
Governor of alabama

Chicago 60637 Ill Illinois
1/9/65

Hon mr George Wallac of the state of alabama
me and other that are concern have Ben writing to
Corrallton ala Pickin for the past 3 or 4 year with
out any sucell at all concern the estate of mr
Edwin Dancy of Dancy ala we wrote to honable
Judge Harris and honable judge mr Hobert H Kirkssey
and honable Judge Kirksey advise me to write the
following names hon. C. G. Robinson Jr   corrallton ala
                  hon. J H curry   alicville ala
                  hon. P m Johnston   gardo   ala
                  hon. N. w Elmore   Reform   ala
                  hon. mrs. Elrod   gardo   ala
                  hon. Hill pate   corrallton ala
                  hon. Ray Kelley

and I wrote to → hon R. G. Robinson — august 25 1964 no
answer and I write again about sept. 15 no answer I feel
that we are in title som consideration by this time
Thank you for what ever consideration your con sine o hase

Dallas Jackson — 1539 E 63 nt
Chicago 60637 Illinois

chicago Ill Jackson Dillon

Mr umbert s. aiello

Mr aiello in Reference to you letter of answer to
My letter of July 29-1964 we have Ben trying to
Get the ProBerty of Mr edward Dancy known
on you Record as Ed win c Dancy Since 1959
the county of Pickens the state of alaBama has
not ask any questions as to who we are are nothing
to try to correct this matter I first Judge Harris
in stead of sending what ever the Record say
he said send him to more information so he
could make out the Record Clearly I then he said
there was no Judge setting at Carrolton ala
Pickens county at that time I then he told atty
Philips mckin that the Recard was Destroyed
By fire in 1874 I and my Brother Edward
Jackson got another lawyer to write and a fee
of $4.00 was Requested and the will was
sent I Gineing the Date of November 8- aD-1889

Book of wills A Page 186, 187
                        188, 189, 190, 191, 192, 193

Dated oct 3-1961
RB Harris   we wants to no why Judge Harris
                 Tell atty Philps mckin the Recard
was Destroyed in 1874 and sent atty Folks a will Dated
1889 which is 14 or 15 years later from 1874

it a Pros to us the this is a case ares looking
the Record to are [3] three lawyer hone how the will
that was sent By Judge Harris and it's some wrong
the Record was Burn By fire in 1874 and a will
was made in 1889 — Contöing [3] page 191. 192-193.
atty Philip s makin wrote for the other pages to as 3 times
But he said the Judge would not send them and he
ask was the will Ever ProBated if so send him
the ProBate no and he again said the Judge would
not send the ProBate nomees the will shows mr
Edward Dowg Requested his wife mrs [an] hassie Dowg
and a Daughter [mis] Sorak ElisaBeth hove theis shore
for the Rest of ther natural life and the heirs
of his side Shall hove ther share the Rest
of theis natural life he supose to hone Died
around 1891 in July are summer My Brother
Edward talk to the NAACP. about it and
they said they under stand a court are supose
to straiten things like this out with any com
twingimt to p leod that [it] look like Predice
Casl to them that some one hone Dis lowerd
that w I are colored and is not interested in
it
                    Dallas J rokson
                    15 39 Eost 63 Rost
                        chicoss ill

STATE OF ALABAMA

GOVERNOR'S OFFICE

MONTGOMERY

GEORGE C. WALLACE
GOVERNOR

January 20, 1965

Mr. Dallas Jackson
1539 E. 63rd Street
Chicago, Illinois 60637

Dear Mr. Jackson:

    This will acknowledge receipt of your letter of
January 9, 1965.

    I read your letter thoroughly and regret that
I cannot be of assistance to you. Unfortunately the
duties of my office are so numerous that I would not
have time to investigate this matter personally and
because of pressing duties my staff is also unable
to help you with this matter. I suggest that you
retain an attorney to investigate this matter and
then advise you concerning your best course of action.

    With best wishes, I am

Sincerely yours,

George C. Wallace
Governor

GCW/ser

October 7, 1963

Justice Department
Washington 25, D.C.

Gentlemen:

    Enclosed herewith please find the following letters, and Documents:

One Will of Edwin C. Dancy, three pages.
One letter dated March 3, 1961 to the County Clerk in Montgomery Alabama.
One letter dated July 6, 1962, to Rev. John H. Jackson at 2601 Waits Street
Gary 3, Indiana, from Mrs. Margaret S. Searcy.
One letter dated August 17, 1962, to Rev. John H. Jackson at 2601 Waits
Street, Gary 3, Indiana from Mrs. Margaret Searcy.
One letter dated October 26, 1959 to Lawyer Wilson at 9115 So. Stewart,
Chicago, Illinois from Gilbert W. Bowles, Tax Collector, Pikens County.
One Death Certificate for Preston Dancy, from the State of Mississippi.
One Census record for Preston Dancy dated January 8, 1963, Census of 1880.
One Census Record for Edward Jackson, dated October 5, 1961 Census of 1920.
One Photostatic copy of a Census Record for Dallas Jackson, dated January
29, 1942, Census of 1920.

                              Very truly yours,

Enclosures: 9

C O P Y

PHILLIP S. MAKIN
Attorney at Law
77 West Washington St.
Chicago 2, Illinois
An 3-3312

March 3, 1961

Clerk, County Court, Carrollton
                  County
County Seat
Carrollton County
Alabama

Re: Estate of Edward C. Dancy,
    Deceased

Dear Sir:

It will be appreciated if you could advise the
undersigned whether or not an estate involving the above-
nemde decedent was ever probated or otherwise administered
by your court.

The named decedent died in Dancy, Alabama approximately
a hundred years ago. If you can find no record of such an
estate in your county court records, will you please advise
me what other court of competent jurisdiction might have
handled it, so that an inquiry could be directed thereto.

I enclose a self-addressed, stamped envelope for your
convenience, and trust that you will oblige. If there is any
fee charged for services requested of you, the undersigned will
be pleased to pay same after notice.

Thanking you in advance for any assistance you may render,
I am

Very truly yours,

s/ Phillip S. Makin

psm;ld
Encl.

March 7, 1961

Dear Sir:

All records of Pickens County were destroyed by
fire 1874. I am confident there is no record
since that date that would involve this estate.

s/ R. B. Harris, Judge of Probate

2009 N. Upland Street
Arlington 7, Virginia
August 17, 1962

Rev. John H. Jackson
2601 Waite Street
Gary 3, Indiana

Dear Rev. Jackson:

On receipt of your letter of July 12, I contacted the Judge of the
Probate Court, Pickens County, Alabama to secure the marriage record
of Preston Dancy and Edwin C. Dancy.

The Judge advises that marriage records prior to 1876 were destroyed
when the Court House burned. Preston Dancy did not marry in Pickens
County, Alabama after 1876.

The 1850 census of Pickens County, Alabama, did not list Edwin C.
Dancy.

The 1860 showed only the following:

> Page 808, Southern Division, P.O. Fairfield, taken 2o & 21, 1860
> Dwelling 499, family 499
>
> EDWIN C. DANCY, aged 49, farmer. He owned real estate valued
> at $13,300, and his personal estate was $45,500. He listed
> his birthplace as North Carolina
>
> No family was shown in the census listing.

Could this be the interim between death of Sabre and Dr. Dancy's second
marriage. Even so, I do not understand not finding them in 1850.

The death certificate of Preston Dancy should show date and place of
birth as well as the names of his parents. You probably know where he
died. So, I would suggest that we secure a copy of his death certificate
and check the 1850 census for the place of his birth. Possibly, Dr. Dancy
did not come to Pickens until after 1850.

Sorry we are running into so much trouble. Let me know where Preston Dancy
died and I'll be glad to attend to getting the certificate for you.

Sincerely,

(Mrs.) Margaret Searcy

Research........$5.00

UNITED STATES DEPARTMENT OF JUSTICE

WASHINGTON, D.C. 20530

Address Reply to the
Division Indicated
and Refer to Initials and Number
A-5-1

April 10, 1967

Mr. Dallas Jackson
6218 South Vernon Avenue
Chicago, Illinois, 60637

Dear Mr. Jackson:

This acknowledges your letter of March 30, 1967,
addressed to the Attorney General.

The matter about which you write is not one coming
within the jurisdiction of the Department of Justice.
In your letter, you stated that you have the services of
an attorney. If you believe he is not handling your case
properly, you may take it up with the Grievance Com-
mittee of the State Bar of Illinois, 10 LaSalle Street,
in your City.

Your enclosures, including a copy of a death record
and a Census Bureau record, are returned.

Sincerely,

Ernest C. Friesen, Jr.
Assistant Attorney General
for Administration

Note A-5-1

UNITED STATES DEPARTMENT OF JUSTICE

WASHINGTON, D.C.

Address Reply to the
Division Indicated
and Refer to Initials and Number

20530

(A-5-1)

October 16, 1963

Mr. Edward Jackson
5422 South Prairie
Chicago 37, Illinois

Dear Mr. Jackson:

Your letter of October 8 has been referred, with
the enclosures, to Mr. W. Neil Franklin, Chief,
Diplomatic, Legal and Fiscal Branch, National Archives
and Records Service, Archives Building, Washington, D.C.,
for consideration.

Sincerely,

S. A. Andretta

S. A. ANDRETTA
Administrative
Assistant Attorney General

2009 N. Upland Street
Arlington 7, Virginia
August 17, 1962

Rev. John H. Jackson
2601 Waite Street
Gary 3, Indiana

Dear Rev. Jackson:

On receipt of your letter of July 12, I contacted the Judge of the
Probate Court, Pickens County, Alabama to secure the marriage record
of Preston Dancy and Edwin C. Dancy.

The Judge advises that marriage records prior to 1876 were destroyed
when the Court House burned. Preston Dancy did not marry in Pickens
County, Alabama after 1876.

The 1850 census of Pickens County, Alabama, did not list Edwin C.
Dancy.

The 1860 showed only the following:

> Page 808, Southern Division, P.O. Fairfield, taken 2o & 21, 1860
> Dwelling 499, family 499
>
> EDWIN C. DANCY, aged 49, farmer. He owned real estate valued
> at $13,300, and his personal estate was $45,500. He listed
> his birthplace as North Carolina
>
> No family was shown in the census listing.

Could this be the interim between death of Sabre and Dr. Dancy's second
marriage. Even so, I do not understand not finding them in 1850.

The death certificate of Preston Dancy should show date and place of
birth as well as the names of his parents. You probably know where he
died. So, I would suggest that we secure a copy of his death certificate
and check the 1850 census for the place of his birth. Possibly, Dr. Dancy
did not come to Pickens until after 1850.

Sorry we are running into so much trouble. Let me know where Preston Dancy
died and I'll be glad to attend to getting the certificate for you.

Sincerely,

(Mrs.) Margaret Searcy

Research........$5.00

OFFICE OF THE CLERK
SUPREME COURT OF THE UNITED STATES
WASHINGTON, D. C., 20543

April 8, 1966

Mr. Dallas Jackson
6134 South Kinbark Avenue
Chicago, Illinois 60637

Dear Mr. Jackson:

In reply to your recent letter addressed to the Chief Justice, I am sorry to have to inform you that the Court is unable to assist you in the matter which you present.

By law, the Court is limited to the consideration of cases brought before it from lower courts in accordance with federal law and the rules of the Court, and it is not possible to give advice or assistance, or to answer questions, on the basis of correspondence.

I am sorry that we cannot be more helpful.

Very truly yours,

JOHN F. DAVIS, Clerk

By J. Osborn
Assistant Clerk

Chapter 2

O ne day in 1929, my 14-year old mom took her personal things to the fields. Years later, my Uncle Elizah said that when his family looked up, my mom had jumped into a wagon driven by my father. Uncle Elizah ran to his parents, shouting, "Dallas stole Gert! Dallas stole Gert!"

My parents settled in Birmingham, Alabama. But when one of my dad's brothers killed a man, they had to get him out of town. That uncle hobo'd to Chicago. Then one by one, each sibling followed— John, Ned, Edward, George, and finally my father, Dallas.

I was only four when we moved to Chicago. Carlton was twenty months old, and Roland was an infant. Two years later, Robbie was born, and two years after that came Dietra. It was then my mom went into postpartum depression and never fully recovered.

We lived in many different apartments on the South Side of Chicago from 29th to 43rd Street. I especially remember living on 36th Street on the west side of Cottage Grove Avenue in the annex of the Vincennes Hotel. The exciting thing about living there was that many black celebrities, like Ella Fitzgerald and the Ink Spots, came to stay while in town. We would all be happy when the Globetrotters came to the hotel.

It was not easy for my father, because there was not a lot of work for Blacks. I vividly remember him applying for employment at a large meat company that was hiring. The receptionist wanted to know why my dad wrote down "Black" for his nationality. He was told, "We do not hire Blacks." But the receptionist took a liking to him as he sat in the waiting room, so she told him to come back in two days but to check the "Caucasian" box that time. Dad did as he was instructed and was hired. Because he had to pass for Caucasian, he had to be on guard about showing family photos.

Dad explained to us that his "passing" was necessary in order to be able to feed us. My siblings and I were too young to be concerned. We just knew, as we were instructed, that should anyone come inquiring about our father, we were to play dumb and refer them to our grandmother.

Every morning when my father would leave for work, he would remind us not to cross over to the east side of Cottage Grove, where there were big private homes. A number of Blacks crossed in an attempt to reach the 31st Street beach; they were beaten or never found.

My family moved within the radius of 29th to 43rd Street so many times that I transferred within the public school system ten times while in grade school. In 1943 my family moved to the newly built housing projects, Robert Brooks Homes, on the west side. There I attended Joseph Medill Elementary and graduated from Joseph Medill High School number one in my class.

We were living on 33rd, two blocks east of Cottage Grove, when I became aware that my mother was very ill. I was eight years old when a police wagon or some county wagon came and took my mom away, kicking and screaming. Dietra was only three months old. Something was very wrong; I did not understand it. As I lay in bed, my eyes were closed, but I was not asleep. I could hear my dad and his sister whispering in low voices. They said my mom had tried to take her own life. My siblings and I were told our mother was ill and was taken to the hospital.

In my little mind, I remembered the man everyone called "Crazy Joe." Joe looked up and talked to the blue sky. He talked to the trees and birds, too. I could not understand why they would take my mother to the hospital in the same manner they did Crazy Joe.

∾

It was at this time they split us up. Roland, Robbie, and Dietra went to live with Uncle Ned (my dad's brother) and his wife, Auntie Sara, who had no children. Carlton and I were sent to live with my father's parents.

My grandparents had applied and were accepted to move into the newly built Ida B. Wells Homes. But they were not allowed to have anyone else move in with them, so Carlton and I were sent to live with Aunt Bertha and her nine children. She did not treat us as well as she did her own children.

Aunt Lena and Uncle Charlie (my dad's brother) lived with their eleven children across the hall from Auntie Bertha. One morning as Auntie Lena saw me leaving for school, she took a look at my messy hair and wanted to know who combed it. When I told her I did, she said I should get up early enough to come to her, so she could comb my hair.

My cousins and I would get together and walk from 29th to 39th to Grandmother's house skipping, running, and jumping all the way. There we would eat cakes, coconut pies, cookies, and candy—all the things children loved.

Grandmother had told the ladies whom she worked for east of Cottage Grove about her motherless grandchildren. These ladies would give her very nice things for us. One lady had a daughter two years older than me and would always give me clothing that her daughter had outgrown.

One Sunday I walked to my grandmother's house to attend church with her. She was very upset that I was not wearing any of the clothing the lady sent me. It was then that Grandmother decided Carlton and I would be moved across the hall to Auntie Lena's. Aunt Lena was saving money to give music lessons to her oldest daughter, Penny. As early as kindergarten I was always singing, and everyone knew I loved music. Auntie Lena, aware of my great love for music, decided Penny would not have her lessons, because she could not afford to pay for both of us.

As I sit here now, my eyes fill with tears when I think of the love that Auntie Lena showed me. She could not have loved me more if I had been her own child. The wings were not there for me to see, but there she was: a real live "angel."

✐

Mom would come home a little longer each time. Finally they thought she was ready. She and Dad had a nice little apartment not far from my grandparents and Uncle Ned. We were to be returned one at a time; Carlton would be first, and I would follow. They wanted to see if Mom could cope with the responsibility. Uncle Ned and Aunt Sara continued to have the responsibility of Roland, Robbie, and Dietra.

Carlton and I were elated to be with our mother. I remember the snow being knee-deep and my father taking us to school, walking ahead and making big steps for us to follow. Christmas came, and we were happy, since we were still with Mom and Dad.

However, Mom's permanent stay was not to be. She soon returned to the hospital. Carlton was born with pneumonia, so my mom always worried about him. Every time they would take her back to the hospital, the last thing she would say would be, "Take good care of Carlton!"

I cannot remember a lot about my mother, but the memory that comes to my mind more than any other is her singing, "Jesus is All the World to Me." She sang this song day after day while she cooked and cleaned. She was an excellent cook and was always baking cakes. On our birthdays she would bake us a cake, and it was our own to do as we pleased: eat it all or share it.

In November of 1941 we were summoned to my grandmother's home and were told our mother had gone to sleep and would not wake up again. She had gone to be with the angels, who would take care of her. I believed from that day that angels were going to take care of me, also. Since that time, God has placed in my path many living angels.

I can vividly remember a time after my mother's death when I was at a crisis point in my life. The owner of my building had wanted my apartment, and after spending days and weeks looking for a place to live, I ended up moving in with my sister. No one wanted children or a single parent.

That morning as I sat in my brother's car as we drove to church. As I looked across the cornfield, I could hear this sweet, melodic voice singing, "All the way my Savior leads me/What have I to ask beside?/ Can I doubt his tender mercy/Who through life has been my guide…"

"Listen! Listen!" I called out.

"Listen to what?" everyone in the car asked.

"Can't you hear it? Can't you hear it?"

No one but me heard anything. When we arrived at church, my brother asked, "What did you hear?" I have always been convinced that the voice I heard was that of my mother's, that her spirit was there to let me know that, if I would let Him, God would lead me out of a stormy period in my life, and all would be well.

❧

A few months after the death of my mother, my father and his sister Mary, a single parent of two, rented an apartment on 33rd and Calumet. The yellow stone building still stands and is one of the buildings in the "gap" that has been renovated. Two years later, my dad left to go on a vacation. Auntie Mary told us that dad was visiting a friend, and when he returned, he would bring with him a new mother.

A week later I came in from school to the rich aroma of cooking. It turned out to be a pot of spaghetti; the smell of garlic, onion, bell pepper and oregano hung in the air.

"You have a new mother in the kitchen, "Aunt Mary explained. I walked in and said, "Hi, Mom. What are you cooking? It smells so good!"

Carlton had stopped outside to shoot marbles. I ran out and called to him, "Carl, Carl! We have a new mom!" He ran into the house and, after looking her over, said, "Hi Mom; I'm hungry." Our new mom laughed, showing her dimples, and replied, "You must be Renee and Carlton. Go and wash up; dinner will be ready soon."

That was the beginning of a beautiful relationship with our stepmother, Mama Eria. We would now be a whole family. But Uncle Ned and Auntie Sara were not willing to give up Dietra. They let Roland and Robbie come to live with us but held on to my little sister. There was going to be a big fight. Mama Eria let it be known that she was told that Dad had five children—two girls and three boys—and she wanted all of them. She was very adamant about getting Dietra, and after a few weeks, Auntie Sara relented.

Shortly thereafter, we moved to the west side. People in the neighborhood did not know that Mama Eria was our stepmother until Mother's Day. She told us to always remember and honor our real mother, and on Mother's Day, she insisted we wear white flowers in memory of our mother. For my siblings and me, Mama Eria wore garments of compassion, hope, understanding, and love. She is and will always be an angel above all angels to us.

At age 13, I became aware that my father was drinking more and spending more time with his brothers and friends. He was also bringing home less and less money. The next year, my youngest brother Elliott was born. At the time of his birth, I was told I had to stay home with my mother, since she was going to have a home delivery with Newberry Center in charge. I cried all day, because I did not want to miss school. I had perfect attendance and wanted to keep it that way. I loved my mother dearly, but until then, can you believe I thought babies came in the doctor's black bag? No one had explained to me the birds and the bees.

As soon as Elliot was old enough, my mother went to work in the Drake Hotel kitchen. Every Sunday she saw that we were in Sunday school. She bought food and clothing and paid the rent, while my dad drank more and more, forgetting us—his responsibility. Each Sunday the brothers would congregate at each other's home and get sloppy drunk. Once they were good and soused, one would designate himself the preacher. Then they would play church, singing one song after the other. They all had very good voices, but they were not able to contain themselves and behave intelligently. Instead, they would clown and make total fools of themselves. Watching them, I vowed I would never, ever drink. To this day, I have not done so.

My dad was a very important person in my life. I hated to see him in a drunken condition. So I thought, "I will do something very good one day, and he will be proud and happy and will not want to drink again." This was an innocent wish of a child who knew absolutely nothing about the power of alcohol.

❧

I graduated from elementary school, sometimes barely making the grade. But in 1944, I entered high school, determined to excel. I wanted my father to be proud and happy. The 1948 *Medillite* shows how I did:

> This June graduating class [...] is one of the most outstanding that has ever been at Medill. Many professions are represented in the aspirations of this class. Either teaching or the textile industry will be more than fortunate to have Renee Jackson as a representative of their field. Renee is the most outstanding graduate, having the highest scholastic rank of her class all four years.

However, high school was not easy due to my voice's soft, high-pitched tone. Whenever I spoke, students would mimic me, labeling me "canary." Many teachers would not let me read aloud, since the class would laugh. In my algebra class, students would go up to the board to write out and explain their problems. When it was my turn, I had to stand aside while the teacher explained my problem for me.

In my sophomore year, I was elected chairperson of the typing staff. It was my responsibility to go to the office each day with a young man to bring the ditto machine to the typing room next door. After several days, Mrs. Press, the school principal, said my voice needed training. She took me inside a walk-in vault and made me say "doo-doooo-doooooo" over and over in as deep a tone as I could. She said that when I came to the office the next day, I was supposed to use my new voice. Every day I would come into the office using my normal voice, and every day she would take me into the vault. After about a week of these "private voice lessons," I told my mother, who was very upset. She went up to the school, and I was never taken into the vault again.

But my voice continued to plague me. When my senior class put on a play, I was given the part of a little girl. At the rehearsal for graduation exercises, Mrs. Press learned that I would give my valedictorian speech. She insisted that Willard, second highest in class, give the speech instead, because my voice was so horrible. Several teachers spoke up, however, and said that regardless of how I sounded, I had worked hard to maintain my grades and had earned the privilege of speaking. Those teachers prevailed.

I won several scholarships, all in the South. However, I felt the need to remain in Chicago to help with my siblings. I was not able to go to college here, so I got a job and helped Mama Eria. Dad was still drinking and had literally turned the responsibility of my siblings over to my mom and me. Mom told me she had considered moving away with me and my siblings, but if I wanted to get married, I should. When I decided to marry Edmond, my childhood sweetheart, she decided at that point to leave my father but to take only her own child.

Dad went into shock when he came home to find our stepmother gone. For the next 44 years until his death, he never touched another drink. My siblings lived with me until each of them finished high school and later married. God took good care of us; my siblings all became professionals with no jail records.

✌

Edmond was tall, dark, and handsome and had personality plus. Any party came alive when he entered the room. He was athletic and liked by all. However, he was also lazy and spoiled. I was 23 years old, but he said I acted like someone who was 43, because I refused to drink alcohol and go to wild parties with him. When our third child was two months old, I found myself taking care of my babies as well as my siblings. With each pregnancy, I worked until I was eight months pregnant. After the third child, I was forced to receive public assistance. Edmond then left and married another girl without bothering to get a divorce from me.

One year later, his mother pleaded with me to take him back. I told her, "My vows meant everything to me and nothing to him. His behavior has shown me that." But she still tried, telling me, "I will pay all the expenses if you promise you will remarry him; give him another chance." "I will not do that," I answered.

His father came to talk to me, also. But he said, "You are a good person, Renee, and are doing an excellent job of caring for your children and your siblings. My son has caused you a lot of pain. He is not ready to be a responsible father or husband. Do not take him back; he will only cause you more pain. My wife would be very upset if she knew I was telling you this. For the sake of my marriage, please do not repeat what I am saying to you. I must say, however, you have a lot of pride—too much pride."

I replied, "I am a poor person. Pride costs nothing, so I can afford to have a lot of it."

My in-laws did many nice things, trying to make up for their son. With three babies, I had many diapers and clothing to wash and needed a washing machine. My father-in-law agreed to co-sign a contract so I could have a washing machine. He went with me to the Good Housekeeping store and selected a washing machine, TV, and new couch. I told him I needed only a washing machine, but he insisted that I get all three. I gave him my word I would never miss a payment and would never cause him any embarrassment. There were many times I did not eat, but I never missed a payment.

Chapter 3

One morning I awoke at 5:00 to the doorbell. The children, my sister, and I were asleep upstairs. My brothers, Roland and Robbie, were sleeping on a sofa bed down in the living room.

An attractive, well-dressed, middle-aged woman stood at the door. She flashed her badge, announcing that she was with the sheriff police. I opened the door.

"Are you Renee?" she asked.

"Yes."

"Open your back door."

I went to open the back door, and there stood a huge man, flashing his badge. The man and I returned to the living room. The lady asked, "Who are these men?" "Ask them," I replied, "They can speak for themselves." When they told her they were my brothers, she asked to see identification.

Satisfied that they were who they said they were, she and the man proceeded to look in all the closets, under the beds, in the refrigerator, and in the cabinets. Once they finished, the lady explained, "It has been reported that a man—your husband—lives here." I responded, "No man lives here—only my children and I. On weekends, my sister and brothers are here." They thanked me for being cooperative and left. I felt very humiliated.

Approximately two months passed, and then one afternoon about 2:00, they returned and went through the same procedure. The children were upstairs taking their noon nap; I was in the kitchen washing and preparing dinner. This visit came about four days after I received my monthly check. The two of them thoroughly checked the cabinets and the refrigerator.

As they were leaving, the lady said, "I am pleased with my finding so far, but you are still under investigation." I did not know why they were coming. I only knew it made me feel very bad.

Three months passed before they came again. This time it was 1 AM. My brothers were asleep downstairs. The two did their usual search, and then the lady admitted, "There is no evidence that a man lives here—no clothing, no shoes, and no male toiletries. I could lose my job for sharing information with you. So if you repeat anything I tell you, I will deny it." She then showed me a copy of the marriage certificate of my husband and another girl. The same judge at City Hall that married us had performed the ceremony for them.

The lady said she had visited the home where my husband was living. She had asked the girl's parents if Edmond had ever spoken of someone named Renee. They told her that he had said that I was his sister and our children were his nieces and nephews. She then showed me a letter reporting me to the public assistance agency. It had the signature of one of my husband's relatives. With my monthly check, I was able to pay the rent and feed my children, signs of independence and the ability to cope with the situation. I can only assume a false report was sent to the agency by my mother-in-law in hopes that I would become dependent on them again and take my husband back.

The lady continued, "I admire you. You are doing an excellent job of caring for your children. No matter when I come, I always find you at home, busy or asleep. I want to give you some motherly advice. You are young. You will marry again. Get yourself a good boyfriend, someone who will be good to you and your children. Keep your business to yourself. Good luck to you, and remember, if you repeat what I've said, I will deny I ever said it."

✐

When my husband married without getting a divorce, my mother-in-law encouraged it but later regretted it. She died never knowing that I knew how she hindered my husband to grow up and be a man.

Edmond was always taking his new girlfriends to meet his mother. Finally she told him, "Do not bring another girl to this house. Why can't you have a lasting relationship with someone?"

He explained, "When I meet a girl, it's because there's something about her that reminds me of Renee. Once I get to know the girl and find out she has none of Renee's characteristics, I lose interest. I want Renee."

Because my husband's male friends envied him and knew I was struggling financially, one by one they tried to proposition me. Some were old enough to be my father. I would turn them down in such a ladylike way that they would be embarrassed. As a result, they had great respect for me and tried to show it.

✐

Three and a half years later, my aunt asked me to attend an affair she was invited to, so I went. There was a young man there, an alumnus from Medill. He was no stranger to many of the people there. His name was George Gerald, but he went by GiGi. He was very handsome, well liked, and popular. All the girls and ladies were interested in him.

All during the affair, he rarely took his eyes off me. When I looked in his direction, he would stare at me until I looked away. Then the tempo of the music changed to a tango, and he came over and asked me to dance.

"I do not dance," I replied, laughing.

"That's okay," he responded, "I'll teach you."

"Really, I do not dance."

"Come—I will teach you. Just follow me."

"Go!" Aunt Paula prodded, "Let him teach you."

Once we were on the dance floor, Gigi gave me instructions: "When I move my right foot forward, move your left foot back. Follow the same procedure with the right foot. If I take your hand to spin you around, make a complete circle." He moved with grace, and I was surprised at my own performance, since we were not allowed to dance when I was growing up.

After the dance, Gigi exclaimed, "You said you did not dance!"

"I do not. I just followed you."

"What is your name?"

"My name is Renee."

"Thanks for the dance, Renee. You did quite well for someone who does not dance."

He did not say anything else to me that night, but he never stopped watching me. Two weeks later, Aunt Paula, who lived two doors down from me, saw him walking down our block, even though he did not live in our neighborhood. Several weeks later, he saw Aunt Paula walking in the neighborhood and asked her for my phone number. She told him she could not do that. However, she said that usually every evening after dinner, I walked my children around the playground.

At least two or three times a week when the children and I went for our walk, Gigi would be sitting on a fire hydrant about a hundred yards from my home. He never said anything as we walked by. He would just wave, and I would wave back. When the children and I returned from our walk, he would be gone. This went on for about five or six weeks.

Then one night around midnight, a noise woke me up. Something was hitting my bedroom window on the second floor. I raised the shade to find Gigi standing there, throwing pebbles. I raised the window and told him to stop.

"Come down," he replied, "I want to talk to you."

"I am not coming down. Go away," I answered.

"I will wake up all your neighbors if you do not come. I want to talk to you."

I went downstairs, my brothers asleep in the living room on a rollaway bed.

"Why are you here this time of the night?" I asked Gigi as I went outside.

"I would like to have your phone number. I asked your aunt for it, but she refused. Whenever I see you, you are with your children, brothers, or sister. They are all asleep now. I wanted to talk to you alone."

"Why do you want to talk to me?"

"You fascinate me, Ren. I like the sound of your voice. I like the way you walk. You are so tiny (I didn't weigh 98 pounds soaking wet) and have such big legs. I want to get to know you."

"My name is *Renee*," I said.

"I know that. I've made it my business to know a lot about you. But my name for you is Ren. I will never call you Renee. Please, may I have your phone number? I know it is unlisted."

I decided to give him my phone number, since I was flattered that he showed such interest in me. I wanted to see him again. After thanking me, Gigi said I should go back inside. He would call me soon.

Several days later, he called and said he was sending me a package in a yellow cab. At 6 PM a cab driver rang my bell and stood there with a bushel basket full of groceries. Every Friday at the same time for the next four weeks, a taxi would come and bring me groceries. During those weeks I never saw or heard from Gigi.

On the fifth week, he called and said, "I did not ask you for a grocery list because I did not think you would give me one. So I made my own list for you. But now I will be calling every Friday morning and want you to have a list ready. I would like to send you what you need and what you want."

That was the beginning of many phone calls. He once told me, "I like talking to you, Ren. I like the sound of your voice. There is so much compassion in it."

About five months after we met, he said he wanted to take me to a party to meet some of his friends—old school mates, he said. I had given away all my nice clothes when I had my first child. So the day before the party, Gigi came to the house with a beautiful dress, slippers and a matching bag for me. I had never had a man buy me clothing. He said, "Please, I ask for nothing in return—only that you look like a doll."

The party was nice, the people warm and friendly. They all appeared to be older than me. Once when I was excusing myself to go to the ladies' room, I heard someone say, "She is so young, Gigi. You are robbing the cradle." He replied, "I am only eight years older than her." Someone else said, "No, no. She is a teenager." When I returned to the table, one of the men asked me if I had finished high school. I told him the school, the year, and my age. He gave me a smile and said, "You could easily pass for sixteen."

Gigi came to the house one afternoon as I was teaching my friend Frances how to make clothes for herself and her daughter. Gigi said, "You have never shown me any of the garments you've made. I did not know you could sew well enough to teach someone."

"This is her machine," I explained. "In exchange for using it, I am teaching her. She is doing very well." I showed him several dresses I had made for my sister and my girls. He was amazed. "It sounds like a very good arrangement," he replied. "You both gain something." I had baked a nice cake, so Gigi stayed long enough to have cake and milk, and then he left.

The following week, Gigi came with a beautiful new Singer sewing machine. He said, "It's nice that Frances lets you use her machine, but you need to have your own. You can still teach her." That sewing machine brought many dollars into my house. For the holidays, I would be swamped with sewing for others.

Gigi and I had been seeing each other for more than a year when one evening, a well-dressed, distinguished looking man rang my doorbell and asked for Gigi. When Gigi stepped outside, he went into a rage, saying, "I do not live here, and you know that! If you like living, don't you ever again come here looking for me. I will see you later." He came back inside and continued watching TV, obviously upset and angry. After awhile he said, "Ren, I will call you tomorrow." And he left. He called the next day, but I did not see him for several weeks.

I knew something was wrong but did not know what it was. I shared the incident with Frances, who asked, "Renee, what do you think about the incident?"

"I haven't the faintest idea," I replied. "I just know that I have never seen Gigi angry or upset, and it bothers me." "My sister knows Gigi and some of his friends," Frances offered. "I'll ask her what she knows."

The next week while at my house, Frances said, "Renee, my loyalty is to you, not Gigi. You cannot let him know that I am telling you this. Everyone knows you two are seeing each other. People know that you are very special to him. You know he is a carpenter and butcher by trade. That makes it easy for him to explain why he always has money. But Gigi is a dealer. He has gone to great lengths to keep you from knowing anything about that part of his life. My sister says that some of the ladies who know more about him are still trying to figure out how you, of all people, got him. They say he talks about you all the time. He affectionately refers to you as 'my doll' but is careful not to call your name. However, people in the inner circle know that it's you he speaks of.

"What is a dealer?" I asked.

"I was afraid you would ask me that. You have lived a sheltered life, Renee. A dealer handles drugs."

"You are kidding!"

"No, I'm not. He is good to you, your children, and your siblings. Until he tells you, and I doubt that he will, don't worry about it. I will be in big trouble if it gets out that I've told you this. You must promise me you will not let it be known." I gave her my promise.

It bothered me. There were times when I could not sleep. Several weeks later, Gigi called and said I should get a babysitter, since he wanted to take me downtown to the theater.

On the way home from the movie, he asked, "What is bothering you, Ren?"

"Nothing," I responded.

"I know you too well. Something's bothering you. You know you can trust me. What is it?"

"Who was the man who came to my house asking for you a few weeks ago?" I asked. He hesitated, then replied, "I was hoping you would never ask. I am not at liberty to say who he is or what he wanted. You cannot tell what you do not know. There are some things about me, Ren, that I do not want you to know. For your sake it is best."

A few days later he came to the house, beaming, with a gorgeous engagement ring. Since he knew that my husband had married another girl without getting a divorce, he said, "I want to pay for your divorce. I want you to be my wife. Will you marry me?"

A few months earlier I would have leaped with joy. However, I just looked at the ring, saying nothing.

"What is it, Ren?" he asked.

"What is a dealer?"

He put both hands up to his head and just held it. "You've known for about two weeks, haven't you?"

"Yes."

"I could tell. Ren, the first night I saw you, you won my heart. There was something about you that was different from everyone in that room. You know I love you. Please marry me."

"Gigi, you will have to give up being a dealer for me to marry you. One day you may be on the front page of the newspaper. I cannot bring that kind of embarrassment to my children."

He said, "It is not that easy, Ren. I know too much; I know too many people in high places. Once in, you can never get out. They would kill me first. I never wanted you to know because I know you. I was afraid you would stop seeing me. Please, Ren. I can do so much for you and the children."

I listened with tears in my eyes. My Aunt Paula had once told me, "I know you care for Gigi. You light up like a Christmas tree whenever he is around." Today, however, my eyes were not sparkling. I knew that under those circumstances I would never agree to marry him.

At that point I should have been strong enough to stop seeing Gigi, but I was not. Several months later, I learned I was carrying his child. I was devastated. But when I told Gigi, he was deliriously happy. When I began to cry, he put his arms around me and kept repeating, "Please forgive me, Ren. Please forgive me. You left me no other choice. I do not want to lose you." And so I continued to see him.

Chapter 4

A month before our child was to be born, Gigi pleaded with me again to marry him. But I still refused. I knew nothing of his activities or the people he associated with. I knew only that he was a licensed carpenter and butcher. He never spent a night in my home, and no one ever came looking for him again. I knew that whatever he was doing had not changed. The subject was off limits. We never discussed it again.

❧

My brother Robbie went into the navy in 1956, and now in 1958, he was coming home from Japan to be the best man in Roland and Denna's wedding. When he arrived, he carried a duffel bag filled with Christmas gifts.

"This is for you, Dietra, and this is for you, Renee. This is for you, Edmond Jr., and this is for you, Renee. This is for you, Bev, and this if for you, Renee. This is for you, Aunt Paula, and this is for you, Renee!" For every gift he gave someone, there was one to match it for me. "Now we know who you really thought about while you were overseas," laughed Aunt Paula. We were able to talk Mama Eria into coming to Chicago for the wedding. It was a real happy time for all of us.

❧

I had a decision to make. I needed to get on with my life and get Gigi out of my system. I decided I would move to the South Side near other family members and would tell no one where I was going. Although I told my children, siblings, and Aunt Paula my plans, I did not tell my friend Frances. The bedrooms and bath were upstairs while everything else was on the first floor, so it was easy to start packing; no one would know unless they went upstairs.

I went to the office of my housing development and asked to be transferred to a housing unit on the far south side. When they wanted to know the reason, I told them my physician recommended it because I was under stress and experiencing a lot of headaches. They said an inspector would be out to see my place and if there were damages, they would not allow a transfer. There would be an unannounced visit to my unit.

A man came two weeks later with pad and pen and went over the apartment. He was amazed at how well it was kept and insisted that I had recently painted the place. I told him it was painted four years ago when they sent someone to paint it but that the walls were clean because I kept them clean. The lawn and flowerbeds were neatly trimmed, and the garden in the back was as well kept as the front. When he asked who helped me keep the place so nice, I told him my children did.

He then said to me, "You do not need to move. What you need is a man, some nightlife. Why don't you let me take you out?" He was a very nice looking Black man, old enough to be my father. It made me angry, but I knew not to show it. I replied, "You are here to determine whether or not I can be transferred to another unit on the South Side, not to discuss my personal life." He said, "You are right. I am here to make that decision, and I can tell you now that you are an asset to this community. Each year we get a bonus for having people such as you. No one in the office will check your place and agree to give you a transfer. We are looking for people like you, so come on—when can I take you out?" I said to him, "I appreciate your coming. If you are finished, you may leave."

The next day, I called my social worker, Pullian, a young Caucasian man. He came to see me, and I told him what happened. He responded, "No one has the right to say where you should live because you are on public assistance. I have turned in my resignation, and the last good thing I can do before leaving is to help you move. I became a social worker to help people, but I am not allowed to help where it is needed. Find yourself an apartment on the South Side near your family. Your rent now is $44 a month. Do not exceed $125, and I will see that it is approved. Once that is done, they will not change it. Call me once you have a place. You have four weeks. You are an intelligent young lady and will do well. Good luck."

Exactly four weeks later, my oldest brother and a cousin came at 4 AM while the neighborhood was still sleeping and moved my children and me.

My brother Roland came home on leave from the army and was not happy with where we lived. It was a well-kept two flat, but you had to walk under a viaduct to get to the bus stop. I was not happy with the place, either—especially the location and neighbors.

Five months later, I started burning up with fever at church. My cousin James carried me to the hospital; I was told I had arrived just in time to prevent complications. My temperature was 106 degrees, and I suffered from a severe strep throat. The next day, my sister called Gigi without my knowledge, since both she and Denna, my sister-in-law, were scared to death. Denna kept saying, "Don't you die on us!"

After I was given IV fluids and a prescription for ten days' worth of antibiotics, I was sent home. Later I awoke to the sound of Gigi's voice in the living room. When I walked into the room, he stood up and said, "Why? Why Ren? Why did you run away?"

"I needed to get you out of my system," I answered. "I did not know any other way." I looked down and did not make eye contact as I spoke, something I had never done before.

"Come. Sit down. Look at me," Gigi said. He took my hands and continued, "You can never solve anything by running away. I was devastated when I went to the house and found you and the children gone. No one knew when or where you had moved. Not even Frances. I went to your Aunt Paula with tears in my eyes, but she refused to tell me how to find you. I cried a river of tears for you, Ren."

I began to cry as I answered, "I need to get you out of my system, Gi."

After looking at me with tears in his eyes for a long time, Gigi responded, "Ren, the best way to get over someone is to replace them with someone else. It is the easiest way, but it is not foolproof. You can find yourself tied down with the replacement, yet in love with the person you are trying to get over. Sometimes it takes years to get a person out of your head and your heart. You can find yourself not completely happy and sometimes miserable. I know you love me, Ren. You know I love you. Say you will marry me. Let me take care of you and the children."

"You cannot give up being a dealer, Gi. I cannot marry you."

"You and I should be together, Ren. You know I would not lie to you. Can't you understand? They will kill me."

He stared at me the way he did the first night he saw me. I cried even more. He then stood up and paced the floor. After awhile he sat down and said, "You are the mother of my child. Please let me buy a home for you and the children. I have the money; it can be done without any ties to me. I'll give the money to one of your brothers to do it."

"No! No! I cannot do that," I replied.

He just stared at me and shook his head. "Will you at least let me help you find a better apartment?"

"Yes. You can do that."

I could not live in a home that was purchased with money that was destroying people. The money he earned as a butcher or carpenter he could spend on us, but I wanted nothing from his other life.

Carlton, home from the army, went apartment hunting with me, and I was able to find a nice apartment a half block from Ogden Park. Carlton and Gigi painted, and Gigi refinished the hardwood floors. It was a very nice apartment with beautiful oak cabinets and woodwork throughout the place.

I told one of the ladies that owned our old place that I would be moving. She replied, "We did not want to rent to you because you have children, but we decided to take the chance. We have watched you close. Your children are well trained, we must acknowledge. We admire how you care for them. You will be a good tenant wherever you go. You are a snobbish little thing, but you are a good mother."

Once we were settled, Gigi said he would honor my wish. Although he now knew where I lived, he would not come by unless I called. He kept his promise:

I did not call; he did not come. It was not unusual to go to the mailbox on any given holiday and find an envelope with several hundred dollars and a note that only said, "Holiday for the children—Gigi."

Chapter 5

My brothers Robbie and Roland both came home in 1960, having finished their tours of duty. Robbie had sent part of his allotment check to me each month, saying he did not want to worry about us, but I never touched a penny of that money. Instead, I saved about $3000 for him. When he became upset that I had not used the money, I told him my children were not his responsibility. I felt he would need his money for himself when he came home until he could find a job. Since he needed transportation, he was able to use that money for a down payment on a car.

∾

We were all going to church, a large congregation with many of my relatives. The church is where you go for refuge when you are hurting, discouraged, and in need of moral support. However, I found very little there. I often wondered where the unfailing love they talked about every Sunday was.

At this church, you had to be from a certain family and belong to the right clique. Back in those days, there was nothing for young single women with children. It was always the ministers and their wives or the young married couples. Unless you were an extremely talented single mother, there was no place of importance for you.

At that time I was too young and inexperienced to know that I needed a personal, real relationship with God. It was not for me to be concerned with the attitudes or dispositions of others coming to worship. It would be a full-time job being what God wanted me to be.

A sister church was established in the south suburban area. My brothers Roland and Robbie decided to go there to worship, and I went, also.

✏

One day the children came home crying; they had taken bottles to get the deposit, but someone refused to give it to them. I went there by myself, asked to speak to the proprietor, and demanded to know why they did not give the deposit to my children. The proprietor, a man named Felton, introduced himself and said he did not know my children. When I gave their names, he knew immediately who they were, especially my oldest son, Edmond Jr., who was known in the neighborhood for his baseball skills. He gave the children the deposit and said there would be no problem in the future.

A few weeks later I attended the funeral of a friend. Felton was there and offered to give me a ride home. He lived only a block away from me, and we became friends.

He knew I loved poetry and music. Twice a week around midnight he would call my house and tell me to turn the radio on to Franklin McCormick, who would recite the poem, "How Do I Love You/Let Me Count the Ways." It had become a routine.

Felton said he was heavily in debt and that several ladies were helping him with his bills. He said he could not afford to get into a relationship with anyone.

Around this time Randy started calling me, as well as another young man, James, from a sister church. James knew my family well, and I knew his. My children liked his great personality. We dated for seven or eight months, and then James engaged an attorney to start proceedings for my divorce. A month later, he came to the house with a set of rings that were simply beautiful. My children loved James, and I was tired of being alone. So I accepted his ring.

I went to see Felton at his place of business to tell him I had accepted an engagement ring. He replied, "You're joking." I responded, "I'm not joking. I will not be calling you, and you are not to call me."

Felton was working on a car. I laid my left hand on the hood next to his, and when he looked down at the ring, his knees buckled. I think he would have fallen, had the car not been there.

While waiting for the divorce, I began to notice that James' fun-loving behavior had turned to a quiet nervousness—almost a depression. The day the divorce papers came with a court date, my brother Carlton told me, "I cannot wait to see James' face when he gets the news. You know, Renee, he is really excited about marrying you."

I replied, "You must not tell anyone that I have these papers. No one must know where I am the day I go to court."

"Why? Why not?"

"I just sense something is wrong and feel led to keep it to myself for awhile."

He promised he would tell no one.

Around this time I was preparing to attend a church convention with my dad and his new wife, Mattie. My luggage was half-packed when my friend

Doris came by and pleaded with me to go with her and a friend to a church lawn party. I decided to go.

Once we arrived, I sat not far from a little old lady who soon called me to sit by her side. I obeyed. She looked at me and said, "You are not to know my name. God sent me here to speak to you. You are a good, kindhearted, easygoing person. But many people take advantage of your kindness. You are at times tempted to strike back. You are the person God meant you to be. Let him fight your battle.

"There are two men wooing you. Run for your life; neither man is for you. One has a habit." (She made a fist and shook it as if she were throwing dice, indicating a gambler. I knew she meant Randy.) "Also, you are going on a trip very soon and have already begun to pack."

By now I could not take my eyes from hers. She continued, "Your income will increase by forty dollars very soon. You will move; I see a green picket fence. I also see you signing your name over and over, and because of it, you will be able to live comfortably. Do not misunderstand me: you will not be rich. But God will bless you far above what you've ever imagined. Stay sweet. Do not change. Do not ask my name, and do not try to find me later. I will not be found."

I sat speechless, my little eyes wide. I knew that only God knew His plans for me, but everything this little lady said about my present circumstances was true. She spoke of my future; how could she know? How could she be so precise?

As we were all leaving, Doris and her friend asked, "Who was that lady talking to you? You had such a strange look on your face. What did she say?" I shared with them everything that she told me. They immediately went back inside the church and said to the little lady, "Talk to us the way you talked to Renee." She replied, "God sent me here to speak to her. I have nothing for you."

❧

Weeks after that, James came to the house, drunk. I had not been aware that he ever drank. When I asked why he was drinking, he started crying uncontrollably. I did not know how to handle the situation and told him he must not let the children see him crying. Carlton, who was there, took the children and went to the park.

James finally calmed down enough to tell me his sisters called him to their home. "They do not want me to marry you," he explained.

"They did not just tell you that today," I replied.

"No. They said they did not think I was serious until I bought the rings. I thought they would be happy for me. Renee, you represent everything my mother ever told my brothers and me to look for in a wife. I do not understand why they are so upset!"

"It's because of my children, isn't it?"

"Yes! But what has that got to do with anything? I have two children, and they want me to marry the mother of my children. I do not want to marry her; I will *not* marry her."

Carlton and the children returned from the park. I asked my brother not to leave, because I wanted to talk to him once James was gone. But when it time came for James to go home, he refused. He kept saying, "This is where I belong. I will not leave!" Carlton responded, "Let him stay tonight. I'll stay, also."

The two of them slept in the living room. I did not sleep well. Early in the morning, I heard James talking with Carlton and then leave for work on the railroad, telling my brother to tell me he would call.

While we had breakfast, Carlton asked, "Why don't you tell him you have your divorce and get it over with?"

"I am not going to marry him," I responded.

"Why not?" my brother asked, very shocked.

"I do not wish to marry into a hostile family. I do not want that for my children."

Several days later, I told James we should not see each other for a while and that maybe he was in love with what I represented to him. Marriage was very serious. We agreed we would not see each other for six weeks.

He came the next day, just long enough to give me an envelope. He said I should keep it where I could see it at all times. Since I did a lot of sewing, he told me to keep it on the sewing machine and that I should not open it until we agreed to see each other again.

When he left, I opened the envelope. Inside lay two needles tied together in the shape of a cross with what looked like straw and weeds. I immediately carried it to the alley and threw it in the garbage can.

The next day I called his mother, who had always spoken well of me to others. I said, "I don't know how to say this to you, but I must, because I love you and care for your son. I believe James has suffered a nervous breakdown." I then told her about his behavior and the envelope he had given me.

"Did you open it?" she asked.

"Yes."

"What was inside?" she asked. I told her.

"And what did you do with it?" she continued. I told her.

I did not tell her about his crying episode or that I was aware her family did not want him to marry me. She was quiet and thanked me for the call.

I did not hear from James, but two months later, I received a call from his mother, who said, "I have bad news. You were right about James. He went to his job and was found wandering around the railroad tracks in his pajamas. He has been in the hospital for three weeks now and is asking for you. Will you come with me to see him?" I replied, "If his doctor approves, then yes, I will come."

James was all smiles when he saw us. We greeted with the usual cheek-to-cheek hug. But he then said, "Renee, I want you to run away with me." I responded, "We will talk about that when you come home. For now, our concern is for your health."

We visited for about thirty minutes. As we were leaving, he said again, "Renee, you and I are going to run away. I have it all planned." "We will talk about it," I replied. His mother listened and thanked me for coming. On the way home, I told her I did not think it would be wise for me to visit him again so he would not think about running away.

When James came home, we did have a long talk. We agreed he should try being reconciled with the mother of his children. I told him he should take the beautiful, expensive rings in case he decided to use them, but he said, "I bought the rings for you. I cannot take them and give them to someone else. Besides, if you and I do not get married, you will always remember me!" I still have the rings today.

Several months later, a close relative came to me and said, "James was shot in his home, and he died. I knew you would eventually learn of this from someone in the church. I needed you to hear it from me." James had already been buried for weeks. I found it painful that his family would bury him and never say a word to me.

I never spoke to his mother again. She died soon after that.

Throughout all of this, I constantly remembered the little old lady. I never saw her again. I didn't even know where to look for her.

Chapter 6

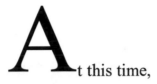

A-t this time, a church convention was going on out of state. Most of the parishioners went, so I was asked to lead worship that Sunday. I asked God to help me prepare, since I had never served in this capacity before. I asked the pastor for the subject of his sermon and then searched for songs that would coincide with the sermon. I was very nervous that Sunday but felt I had done as well as those who were worship leaders all the time.

However, people later asked, "Why was *she* doing the devotion? Who gave *her* permission?" as though I was unworthy to lead the congregation in hymns and praise. It was very painful to hear this. I did not say anything, but I lost all desire to ever serve in that capacity again. I began to spend more and more time with those who did not attend church. They were more sincere and did not wear false faces.

✌

1961 came, and along with it a call from Gigi. He said he was getting married and had purchased a home not far from where I attended church. He wanted me to have his phone number in case I needed him. He said he had told his fiancé about me and Gamal, our son. It would be okay to call, he explained. I listened as he gave me the number, but I did not write it down. He would soon be a married man. I would never call his home, and Gi never called me again.

As I started going to church less, I renewed my friendship with Randy. Seeing him was not about love or commitment; it was just something to do. I was young and not committed to birth control, so my youngest son Gregory was conceived in the heat of the moment. When I told Randy, he suggested I get an abortion. I did not agree, so that ended whatever there was between us.

I found it difficult to find words to even try to describe the relationship between Randy and me. Reflecting back now, I can only say that out of loneliness, disappointment, and rejection, I turned to Randy for solace.

By the time Gregory was one year old, Randy wanted very much to renew our friendship. But I was not interested. I wanted no part of him ever again. While pregnant, I learned that there were many women in Randy's life. I was thankful to be able to escape with my *own* life. I did not wish to be part of the parade.

People I knew outside the church were warm and loving and showed great concern for me. Except for shoes, I did not buy any clothing for Gregory until he was two years old. As an infant he wore the best, and none of it cost me a dime. While carrying him, I often thought of the little lady telling me to run for my life.

✌

About this time, Uncle Jim, one of my dad's brothers, became seriously ill and was not expected to live. However, God was good to him, and he survived. When the time came for him to be discharged from the hospital, he had nowhere to go, so I let him come with me, the children, and our cousin Katie. By now my brother Robbie was married and no longer lived with us.

I went to the Social Security board and got Uncle Jim's benefits started, but his allotment was meager. He thanked me for taking him in and wanted to know how much I would charge. I said I wanted nothing, since he would need money to get his own place when he was stronger. When I said he would need to contribute towards food, he asked if forty dollars would be sufficient. I agreed. Again, I thought of the old lady.

ᴈ

During this period, I often found myself in the "Valley of Baca," weeping. I missed church but lacked the courage to return. Usually my tears came in the late night or early morning; I did not want my children to see how I cried until there were barely any tears left.

I knew about salvation but did not know about having a real, personal relationship with God. Still, I longed to be in His presence. I kept my Bible open on the 84th Psalm and read it often, finding strength in its words. I knew that Joy would come in the morning. In God's morning of my life.

How amiable are thy tabernacles,
O LORD of hosts!

My soul longeth, yea, even fainteth
for the courts of the LORD:
my heart and my flesh crieth out
for the living God.

Yea, the sparrow hath found an house,
and the swallow a nest for herself,
where she may lay her young,
even thine altars, O LORD of hosts,
my King, and my God.

Blessed are they that dwell in thy house:
they will be still praising thee. Selah.

Blessed is the man whose strength is in thee;
in whose heart are the ways of them.

Who passing through the valley of Baca make it a well;
the rain also filleth the pools.

Psalm 84:1-6, 10

One day when I went to the mailbox, I found a letter from Minister Dora Cobb, one of the mothers of our church. While reading her words, I could feel her love and compassion for me. I kept the letter for many years until it turned yellow, ragged, and worn. Whenever I felt low in spirit or depressed—and there were many of those days—I would read her letter. Although I would always cry whenever I read it, I would draw strength from her words. In essence, she wrote:

> I love you and would like to be available to you. You are a very sweet young lady. I hope these words will be of solace to you. God loves you and forgives you every day. He did not make any perfect human being. Before you were born, women young and old were making the same mistakes, looking for love in all the wrong places. They will be making these same mistakes when you are dead and gone.
>
> I want you to hold your head up high and continue to be the sweet person God has made you to be. God loves and cares for you. I love you too. Do not hesitate to call me day or night, if you feel the need. I would love to see you back in church. I will be remembering you in my prayers.

Weeks later I called and thanked her for her letter of love. I told her that whenever I felt bad, I read her letter. I also promised her I would come to church soon.

A month later I made the decision to return to church. I went with my mind made up that nothing anyone did or said and that no inclusion or exclusion would cause me to leave again.

Six months after my return, Mother Cobb told me she was growing old and needed someone to take her place on the ordinance board for serving communion. I had felt looked down upon by numerous people, even in the small church. I could not believe she wanted to teach me to serve communion. But she took me under her wing and taught me what to do. I considered it an honor to assist her. What greater honor could there be than to prepare the Lord's Supper?

I have done so from that day until this. For 35 years I have prepared communion with love in my heart for every partaker. Mother Cobb's letter meant so much to me. It is my desire to walk in her footsteps. I want to be a blessing and encouragement to other young women. My eyes fill with tears of gratitude even now, as I remember the compassion and love shown to me by this gentle, soft-spoken woman.

Now that I have grown in my relationship with God and the Holy Spirit, I am mature enough to know that I cannot blame the people in church for the bad choices I made. God gives us free will. It is up to us to choose wisely. Because of my experiences in the church, I ask God to give me a double portion of love, compassion, and understanding to give and to share— not only with everyone I meet, but especially with those who enter the doors of our church.

In the past I was depending on my own strength. I was going to church and working in church but did not have a close relationship with the Holy Spirit. I now know that it is impossible for me or for anyone to be in the will of God without the indwelling of the Holy Spirit. When the Holy Spirit is alive in you, not only will you know that God is alive in you, but everyone who comes in contact with you will know, also. The Holy Spirit cannot be contained but flows over to others.

Mother Cobb wore the garments of an angel!

Chapter 7

I t was in 1967 that the phone rang and a young lady on the other end asked to speak to Gigi. I said, "You have the wrong number. No one lives here by that name."

"May I speak to Ren?" she then asked.

"I am Ren."

"I am Jean, Gigi's wife. We had a big fight, and he left home four days ago. This is the first time he has been gone four days. I *know* he is there with you. When he left, he told me he would always love you. I *know* he is there!"

"What makes you think he is here?" I asked.

"At times he speaks of you unceasingly," she replied, crying. "I feel like I know you. Sometimes he has even called me by your name. I don't even know why he married me. He has never stopped loving you!"

"Where did you get my phone number?" I asked.

"It's in our phone book."

"Is the address there?"

"No."

"I have not seen Gigi since 1958. The last time I spoke to him was two weeks before you two were married. He called and gave me your phone number, but I did not write it down, because I did not plan to call. That was about four years ago. I have never dated a married man and do not plan to do so. I am sorry you are having problems and do not want you to agonize, thinking he is here. Get a pencil; let me give you my address. You have my permission to come unannounced day or night and see for yourself, if it will make you feel better. But you will not find him here."

She had stopped crying and was very quiet. When she spoke, she said, "Thanks for the invitation. I can now understand why he loved you."

"My invitation is genuine. You may come any time you like."

She never came to see for herself.

∾

Around 1968, the owner of our building came home from the service after a tour of 20 years. He needed my apartment for his family and only gave me 30 days to find an apartment for myself. He said mine was the best-kept apartment in the building, since the beautiful woodwork had not been painted over. Also, the landlord said he did not want any children in his building.

The real estate agent told him he should ask one of the other tenants to move and give me that apartment, because my children and I had taken care of his building without pay. My boys cut the grass, and I attended the furnace and kept the foyer clean. I did so because I took pride in where I lived. It did not matter to me that I did not own the building. Dietra, who had moved in on the first floor, would tell me I was crazy when I mopped the foyer. "Let them pay a janitor," she would say. Children lived in all four apartments in the building: apartment one had one child, two had two, and three had three. But I had five children; we were not wanted.

I had to look for a place to live. The little lady had said I would move, but I had not believed her.

I moved to 79th and Sangamon. Cousin Katie had gone to live with her sister, Gregory was ready for kindergarten, and I was ready to return to school, so that I could become self-sufficient and not be a burden to my children in my old age.

Dad wanted me to take up beauty culture and work in the shop with him and his wife. But when times are hard, people do their own hair. Since I wanted a steady job, I decided on nursing.

I took the National League of Nurses test and scored high. After buying books and uniforms, I called my social worker, Mr. Sherman, and told him my plans. He replied, "You are an intelligent young lady and will do well. I will see to it. You will have extra money for uniforms, transportation, and a babysitter. I once wanted to be a doctor but could not make the grade. So I will live my dream through you. I ask just one thing: to see all your test papers so I know how you progress."

It was not easy. There were 80 students, 20 in four different hospitals. My first assignment for basics was at Holy Cross Hospital. Out of its 20 students, only four were Black and eight were over 30 years of age.

The teacher (I will call her Ms. Molly) immediately set out to eliminate the Black students. One Black student who was older than me was eliminated in two weeks. I was 32, and the other two Black students were 27 and 18.

Ms. Molly then began to work on me. I learned early on that I would need more than myself to cope with her. Each day before leaving for the hospital, I would ask God to go inside with me and to please not leave me alone. I'd also read a portion of Hebrews 13:5.

"I will never leave thee nor forsake thee."

I would then go to class with great confidence. My book bag was heavy with all my books, but I found room to place a small, white Bible inside. Even though I did not have time to open it, it felt good just having it close by.

We were on the wards every morning and in class every afternoon. Quizzes were given during the week, and our big test was every Monday afternoon. Each Monday morning, Ms. Molly would scream at me so badly I would want to cry. However, I would not give her the satisfaction of seeing my tears. The more she screamed, the harder I prayed.

Despite Ms. Molly's tactic to unnerve me before the test, I always scored 90% or above—often 100%. Soon she knew that just screaming on Monday mornings would not affect my grades, so she'd speak to me so ugly throughout the week.

For example, one morning we were to put in place an indwelling catheter. As another student and I stood at the foot of the patient's bed, the student fainted and fell between the patient's legs. The student was removed, and I was next in line to do the procedure.

Because of all the excitement, I wasn't sure I remembered all of the instructions. I assumed that Ms. Molly would give me all of the directions, then let me do the procedure uninterrupted, as she did for the other students. However, she refused and instead roughly walked me through the procedure one step at a time, which made me jittery. However, I was still able to put the catheter in place.

As we left the room, Ms. Molly screamed, "Renee, what do you use for brains?!" I knew she was trying to set the stage so she could write me up for insubordination and have me dismissed from class.

The morning we were to have our midterm exam, Ms. Molly spoke to me so ugly in the nursing station that one of the physicians turned to her and asked, "Do you have a problem? Why are you talking to that young lady like that? Every morning you scream and holler at her. Why?" Ms. Molly turned red as a beet. She never screamed at me in the nursing station again. Instead, she would catch me down the hall, away from the hearing range of others.

No matter what she said, I would be quiet unless she directly asked me a question. If I raised my hand, she would never call on me. But if I did *not* raise my hand, she would call on me, assuming I did not know the answer. When I would give the right answer, she would look at me a very long time, and then ask someone else the same question. I did not care. She had her nursing degree, and I was trying to get mine.

Once she saw she could not break me, she went to work on Jennifer, the 18-year-old Black woman who was now struggling to keep up her grades. I told Jennifer she needed a study partner and offered to study with her, since I was told I took excellent notes. I shared my notes and told her to write them down at least twice. On Sunday afternoon, I would quiz her to see how much information she had retained. Her grades went up, and her name was taken off the probation list.

The day before leaving Holy Cross, we received our next assignments: both Jennifer and I were scheduled to go to Michael Reese Hospital for Med-Surg. On the last day, we got our evaluations. Jennifer was one of the first to go speak with Ms. Molly. When she came out crying, everyone wanted to know why.

It never occurred to me to tell Jennifer not to tell anyone, especially Ms. Molly, that I was her study partner. Almost everyone had a study partner. But when Ms. Molly asked Jennifer how she managed to pull her grades up and Jennifer told her that I was her study partner, Ms. Molly changed Jennifer's assignment to Cook County Peds. I knew another lady who was scheduled to go to Cook County and later asked her to be a study partner for Jennifer, which she did.

When I went in for my evaluation, Ms. Molly discussed my grades, which were good. Then she leaned back in her chair and said, "I see something in you. There is something about you that is different from anyone in this class. I have not been able to put my finger on it." She sat there and looked very hard at me as if waiting for me to tell her what it was. I sat with my hands folded in my lap and just smiled. I did not part my lips.

When she saw I was not going to respond, she picked up my evaluation and said, "You are always mothering people. I see it as a negative thing, so I am writing it in your evaluation. You do agree that is negative?" "I am a mother," I said—nothing more. I knew what she was referring to. Two of the young Caucasian girls would come to me with their problems, and I would help them, if I could. They had also invited me to their homes to meet their parents.

The rest of my evaluation went well. There was nothing to complain about: my grades were high, and I was clean, on time, and mannerly. As Ms. Molly completed the evaluation, I made no extra conversation, speaking only when required.

Later when one of the other ladies was taking a collection to give Ms. Molly a gift, she told me, "We do not want you to give anything, Renee. We all know she was very mean to you."

❧

My next training was in Geriatrics at a Jewish home. During my last week, I was assigned to two little ladies. One of them watched every move I made. I gave her total care, while she never said anything.

The day before I left, she said, "Young lady, you have *charisma*!" I wore a blank look on my face. She could tell I did not know what she was talking about and asked me, "Do you know the meaning of *charisma*?

"No," I said.

"Can you spell it?" she asked.

"No."

So she wrote the word down for me. "When you come tomorrow, tell me the meaning of this word. You should know the meaning of what you have."

That day the word became part of my vocabulary.

✌

At graduation, all the classes came together. Jennifer struggled but made it. The student with the highest grades would speak; another would present the class gift. The decision was made between a pretty young lady and myself. When I was chosen, the lady cried uncontrollably, saying, "How could they choose her over me?" One instructor said I was chosen since several instructors thought I had good diction.

I began full-time employment at the University of Chicago as a Licensed Practical Nurse. During an eight-hour shift, I would sign my name many times to the patients' charts. I thought about the little old lady.

He is good. He is good.
His mercy endures forever.
He is good.

Psalm 106:1

Chapter 8

A coworker, Shirley, kept bugging me. She wanted to introduce me to a friend of hers. I eventually gave in and said okay.

His name was Haywood. As it turned out, he was dependable and always kept his word. If he was going to be late, he would call. He also planned things that included my children. A divorced man, he wanted me to meet his own children, and I got along well with them. He wanted to be in a committed relationship, and so did I. Haywood, Gregory, and I would go to the movies together. On my day off, we would go for long rides out in the country.

After dating six months, Haywood and I were married at home in a quiet ceremony with our families present. My dad said he had attended many large church weddings but had never seen anyone get as many gifts as me. You could not walk in my 20 x 20 living room due to the gifts. My friends were very generous; I did not buy linen for almost 10 years.

Haywood did not believe in bills. He believed in paying cash for everything, so he had no established credit. I told Haywood I was saving to buy a house; he said his mother needed a car, and he had promised to buy her one. He wondered if I would have any objection, and I told him no. Haywood got paid every week; I got paid every two weeks.

The first paycheck after our marriage, I showed Haywood my check stub. I thought when you get married, you share, and there should be no secrets. Instead, I got my first disappointment. Haywood said, "I do not want to see your check stub, because you will never see mine." I did not know what to say, so I did not say anything. After that, I never brought another check stub home. I left them in my locker.

I was aware that each month a bond was taken out of Haywood's check in his mother's name. But I had no objections, even though his mother and I did not have the best relationship. She told me almost as soon as Haywood and I were married that I should start preparing to move to Arkansas. She said she was getting old and she expected "Son"(as she called him) to come home and take care of her. She said, "You are a nurse. It will be easy for you to get employment here." I replied authoritatively, "It is not for him to uproot me to bring me to you. You must come to me." She was very unhappy about the way I felt and voiced her opinion.

One year after our marriage, we bought a lovely home near 78th and Wolcott. Haywood tore out the back porch and stairs and rebuilt them. He then painted the yard fence green. I thought of the little old lady.

Some of my coworkers were bugging me about going back to school. I was doing RN work but receiving LPN pay. Then there was a fallout in one of the RN classes, and six people were needed as replacements. LPNs could go into the class and skip the first semester if they scored high enough on the exam. I wanted to go back to school, but I wanted to start at the beginning. Whenever Ed Miller, a pharmacist, would come to the floor, he would say, "Did you get yourself registered in school today?"

Haywood also encouraged me to do so. He said, "The door of opportunity has opened. Take it while it is there. They would not ask you to skip a semester if they thought you could not handle it." So I did.

I had quite a load to carry: going to school full-time, working every weekend from eleven to seven, having a home to upkeep and a husband and children to care for. I carried the little white Bible this time for a different reason. However, in 1974, I graduated as an RN and returned to full-time employment.

❧

In July 1975 my daughter, Bette, called me from work. She was a nurse at Northwestern Memorial Hospital and said, "Mom, there is a man here in Intensive Care. He was beaten so badly you could hardly recognize him and then left for dead. Every time I go near his bed, he calls me Ren. The doctors asked if I knew him. I said no. Mom, didn't Gigi call you Ren?'

"Yes," I replied.

"What's his middle name, Mom?"

"Gerald."

"Hold on, Mom, while I check his chart."

She came back to the phone and said, "Mom, the man's name is George Gerald. It is Gigi."

I asked Haywood if he would take me to the hospital to see Gi, but he told me to wait until Friday. When Bette arrived at work on Friday morning, she called to say that Gigi was dead. I felt very bad that I didn't get to see him before he died.

Gamal was in the Army, but the Red Cross sent him home for the funeral, which was a closed casket one. I sat with my son in the back pew; as the family was leaving, Gigi's wife stopped and said, "I knew as soon as I saw you that you were Ren. I knew you would be here if you were aware of Gigi's death. I am glad you came." She then continued to the limousine.

I placed the beautiful diamond that Gi gave me in a necklace. One day I will give it to one of Gamal's daughters.

Chapter 9

T he next week, Haywood had a friend pick him up for work at General Motors in LaGrange. He then came home that evening with a new Chevy Caprice for me. Haywood was planning to get me a new car and decided this would be a good time to do it to lift my spirits.

Haywood was a good person, if he liked you. He would give you the shirt off his back. He wanted me to have the best of everything. The problem was that he had a split personality. He could be so sweet one minute and so horrible the next. He also resented anyone with knowledge, since he was not educated.

His mood swings were so severe that once I suggested he see a doctor. He got angry and said, "Just because you've gone back to school, you think you know it all." Years later when he did see a doctor, we learned that a tumor had been growing on his brain for years.

❧

The next few years were rough. My daughter, Bev, lost custody of her six children. My sister, Dietra, took three of them, and I took the other three. Before he left for Germany, Gamal came home on leave from the army. He brought with him his wife, Soon-Na, and their daughter, Lucinda, and left them with me.

Soon-Na was a lovely person, easy to get along with. Everyone loved Soon-Na except Haywood, who was unnecessarily cruel to her. When I was at work, Haywood would have Soon-Na do chores that I would not have her do. He wanted to treat her as though she was a servant, rather than part of the family. I am sure it was because she was of a different nationality. Haywood had low self-esteem; it made him feel big to give orders.

Haywood had a daughter, Alicia, outside his first marriage. Since her mother had a heavy drinking habit, Haywood wanted his older daughter to take Alicia. But I said, "No. One more here will not make that much difference. Bring her here." Alicia and I had a beautiful relationship. She seemed to adore me, and I treated her as if she were my own child. I did nothing for my son Gregory that I did not do for Alicia. However, Haywood was envious of our relationship and often told her she acted like she loved me more.

When Haywood bought the new Chevy for me, the first car bought for me was sold to his first wife for $100. A used car was then bought for his mother. When he bought his first new Cadillac, he gave his old car to one of his daughters. In 1979 he decided to give the Caprice to his mother. It had 35,000 miles, was steam cleaned, and looked brand new. The used car she was driving was then given to his son. He then bought me a Park Avenue and the next year bought his second new Cadillac.

Haywood's Aunt Olivia loved me dearly. When she came to visit every year, she always stayed at our house. This differed from Haywood's mother, who would only stay a day with us and then spend the rest of her visit with Haywood's first wife.

In 1982 on one of her many visits, Aunt Olivia was up having breakfast when I came in from work. She said she needed to talk to me before anyone came home and said, "Baby girl, I am grieved. Your marriage is in trouble. My sister and 'Son' are making plans for the future, and those plans do not include you. Do *not* help him get another car."

She handed me a one hundred dollar bill, saying, "I want you to put this in a bank account and to not tell Son. Every payday, add five or ten dollars—whatever you can afford. You will need it to pay for your divorce!

"I told Son that when I die, he is to sell my property and divide the funds equally with all of the children—yours and his. However, he plans to do something else with it. If I wanted that done, I could do it myself.

"I am eighty-two years old and will not live much longer, so I will be selling my property very soon. I want an address where I can write to you without Son's knowledge." I gave her the address of Carlton, my oldest brother. I was not aware at that point that my marriage was in trouble. I did not have a problem with his mother staying with his ex-wife when she came to visit. I wanted her to be wherever she felt comfortable, She was 80 years old. Besides, her grandchildren were there.

❧

Haywood came home one evening from work and said, "My boss says the nurses in the city make more than nurses in the suburbs. His wife is a nurse, and he said she makes good money." I replied, "Yes, that is true." He wanted to know which hospital paid the most. I told him Cook County was number one, Osteopath was second and the University of Chicago was third. He just stared at me. He was always saying how he brought home the real money and I brought home the peanuts.

The following Friday, Haywood laid his check stub on the kitchen table, hoping I would pick it up. However, I did not touch it and gave instructions to Soon-Na and the children not to do so, either. I remembered the many times he stood at the waste can and tore up his check stubs in my face to keep me from seeing them.

The next morning when he left for work, I dumped the trash on the kitchen floor and recovered every piece of that stub, which he had torn up.

Soon-Na came in and asked, "What are you doing, Mama?" I replied, "You are not to tell Daddy." (She called Haywood "Daddy.") I retrieved at least five stubs on different occasions and put them in my work locker with my own stubs.

I do not know why I did all this, because I took care of all the business that required reading. Since Haywood had great difficulty reading, I took care of filing our taxes. All I had to do was take the figure from his tax statement to figure out his weekly pay. I really cannot say why I retrieved Haywood's torn check stub, except that it was an insult for him to tear them up in my face. God and God only knows why I did that.

Three weeks passed, and Haywood laid his stub on the table again. It stayed there on the table for a week, untouched. Finally, he removed it. I assumed he now wanted to see my check stubs. He obviously had forgotten that it was he who set the rules, and I was going to continue to abide by them. I never showed him my check stubs.

❧

I never objected to anything Haywood would do for his first wife and their adult children; in fact, I tried to show his children the same love I showed my own. But as time went on, Haywood began to spend more time in his first wife's company.

After a dispute one day, Haywood told me, "I think my first wife is ready to take me back now. I don't have to put up with any nonsense from you." "You are not being held here by force," I answered, "You are free to leave at any time."

When Haywood became physically abusive with Gregory, Alicia, and me, I immediately hired an attorney to get a divorce. But since I wanted my marriage to work, I didn't file for divorce right away.

Haywood purchased all his cars through his credit union. The payments were taken before he got his check; thus, he had no established credit. In 1983, when Haywood wanted to buy another car, he was too ashamed to ask for another loan from the credit union, because he had previously cursed out some of their people. I had not even been made aware that he was shopping for a car.

I came home from work one Saturday morning, and breakfast was ready. This wasn't unusual, since Haywood would cook breakfast every weekend that I worked. But on this particular morning, he wanted me to go for a ride with him and would not tell me where we were going.

We stopped at Heritage Cadillac in Lombard. Haywood selected the car he wanted, but when the finance contract was prepared, he could not get the car without my signature. Since I had A-one credit, I signed for the car. It was Haywood's third new Cadillac during our marriage. The car cost $33,000, while our home cost $25,000. Later I called Auntie Olivia and told her I had not been obedient to her. I told her that since I appreciated Haywood allowing me to bring my grandchildren into our home, I felt obligated to help him. She replied, "You are a good mother and wife and are doing your best. I will keep you constantly before the Lord. It will be okay."

Two months later, Carlton called and said I had mail at his house. He said he would bring it to the funeral of Leo, Dietra's husband. When I opened the envelope, I found a cashiers check for $2000 and a tiny piece of paper saying, "I will see you soon." Carlton asked what the money was for; I told him I did not know. He said, "Since she chose not to send it to your house, do not take it home. Come tomorrow, and I will give it to you. Then take it to the bank."

The following week, Auntie Olivia came. She asked, "Did you get the package? What did you do with it?" "Yes, I put it in the account you told me to open," I answered. "Very good," she said. "You will need it to pay your attorney."

Later that same year, there was another dispute. Alicia told a lie, implying that I was lying. I demanded an apology. If Alicia had acknowledged that she was afraid to tell the truth, I would have understood and dropped the incident. Instead, she just flatly refused to apologize, even though her father begged her to do so.

On Saturday morning when I came home from work, I asked her if she was ready to apologize. Haywood said, "She does not feel she has anything to apologize for."

I replied, "My children are older than her, and they give you total respect. I will not settle for anything less from her. She must leave."

As I prepared for bed, I said to Haywood, "When I get up, I want an apology. If I do not get it, I want her out. There can only be one woman here." Before I fell asleep, I heard him pleading with Alicia, "Please tell her you're sorry. Please, Alicia." She stood her ground.

When I got up around noon, they were packing. Haywood told me, "If she has to leave, then I will leave." I replied, "Then that is your choice to make. Do whatever pleases you. Should you leave, please know that you cannot come back."

They packed as many of their belongings that his new car could hold. The next day I called my attorney, then the locksmith to change all the locks, then Auntie Olivia. She said, "My heart is heavy. You are the best thing that ever happened to Son. I believe God was blessing him through you. When he walked away from you, he walked away from his blessings. As soon as I learn where he is, I will call you."

Two days later she called and said, "Your husband is in Waukegan at Vera's. Do you know her address?" I said yes. Three days later Auntie Olivia told me he was back in Chicago. She said, "I will keep up with him for you, since you must keep up with the car."

I later learned that Haywood wanted to get a new car while he was married to me and was then going to stay until Alicia graduated from high school. She had two years to go. He told others, "Renee will give Alicia everything she wants and will take care of all her graduation needs. There is nothing Alicia will need that Renee will not get."

But those were not God's plans for me. The next month, the doorbell rang. A deputy sheriff brought Haywood's petition for divorce. I was not surprised, but I was hurt and angry at all the lies it contained.

Two days later, Haywood's attorney called. I listened as he spoke for thirty minutes. When he finished, I said, "You will find out that your client is a big liar. All those accusations are lies." He said it would be less costly if he represented us both. When I hung up, I called my own attorney, who called Haywood's attorney and told him that he was not to call me. He could not believe he had spoken to me for that long and I never gave any indication I had an attorney.

Two months later, Haywood, Alicia, and his first wife drove to Arkansas in the Cadillac. He became ill, returned, and went directly to the hospital for surgery. A close friend gave me the information, so I went to see him. When I walked in, he said, "I know you. There is no way someone would tell you I was in the hospital and you would not come."

I had received a past due notice on the car. When I handed it to him, he said, "I need you to go to the car dealer and to GM to get some forms for me. I am sure I have insurance that will pay my bills while I am off." But I was not interested in his bills; my concern was the car.

Haywood told me he had surgery for tuberculosis. As a nurse, I knew you do not operate for tuberculosis, because it is treatable. I spoke to the head nurse and was told he was there to rule out lung cancer.

The next day I went to the car dealer and GM, then returned to the hospital. I needed to let Haywood know there was no insurance and that I needed to know his plans for paying the car note.

When I arrived at the lobby desk, the attendant asked my name. When I gave it, I was told I would have to go to security. There I was, looking good in a full-length black mink coat and matching hat, being told to go to security. I was livid! Having been a nurse for a number of years, I knew what that meant: I was barred from visiting.

I told the young man in security who I was and that I had been there the day before when my husband asked me to run an errand regarding his car. I handed him all the papers, including the overdue notice. He then asked to see my identification, which I showed. He read the papers, got angry, and started cursing, saying, "How could anyone have the nerve to bar you from seeing your husband when just seven months ago you signed for his car that cost more than my house! One minute. You are going upstairs, and I have no intention of accompanying you." He went to the phone, and I heard him ask to speak to the head nurse. Then he came back and said, "You may go upstairs."

The elevator stood right in front of the nursing station. When the door opened and I stepped out, everyone stopped whatever they were doing to look at me. I was so embarrassed. I approached the desk and gave my name, and the young lady said I could go to Haywood's room.

Haywood knew I was upset when he looked in my face. I said, "How could you do that to me? Why would you ask me to come here today, knowing I would be embarrassed?"

"I didn't do it. My daughter did. When you were here yesterday, you ran my temperature up."

"You mean I ran your blood pressure up."

"No. My temperature—you ran that up."

"If your temperature went up, it is because you have an infection. It is impossible for me or anyone else to run your temperature up. Listen! And hear me well. You wanted a new Cadillac, not I. If you miss one payment or if I ever receive another overdue notice, I give you my word that I will begin procedures to have that car repossessed. I *dare* you to miss a payment." I walked out and did not look back.

The day Haywood left home, he and I exchanged car keys. He gave me his key to the Park Avenue, and I gave him the keys to the Cadillac. He did not know that the day he sent me to the dealership, they were shocked to learn we were getting a divorce. Since they knew I had co-signed for the car, they asked if I had keys. When I said no, they immediately made me a set. I did not see Haywood again until the day in August when we were scheduled to be in court.

By April I was not happy with my attorney; I could tell she was leaning toward Haywood's attorney's decision. So I dismissed her and got myself another attorney. For the rest of my days, I will remember attorney Shapiro.

In May he called and said, "I am dropping your petition for a divorce. It seems important to your husband that he get rid of you, so we are going to let *him* divorce *you*. Your husband and his attorney want everything sold and divided, and your husband is asking for the organ."

"Oh no! Not my organ."

"Why would he ask for it? Can he or his daughter play it?"

"No."

"Well, for one, it is the most expensive piece of furniture in the house. Two, if you want it bad enough, you can buy it back for a price, and three, that will give your husband money to pay for his lawyer."

I could not believe it. Haywood knew how much that organ meant to me. I said, "I worked two jobs to pay for that organ. I will not buy it from him or anyone else. He can have it. God will provide me with the means to get another one."

"Very good. I was hoping you would say that. It was your decision to make, not mine."

I left Shapiro's office, went directly to Music World, and paid down on an organ even better than the first.

✌

One week before the divorce, attorney Shapiro summoned me to his office. "I have good news," he said, "Remember, we are letting him divorce you. On Friday you are to answer only the questions asked of you. No matter what your husband says, you are to remain silent. Do you think you can do that?"

"Yes."

"Well, here it is: you get to keep your car, the house, and everything in it."

"Everything?"

"Everything. Your husband will keep the Cadillac. He will come on Thursday and remove all his belongings. Unfortunately, we cannot remove your name from the car. It will not be easy for him. We will have to trust God that he meets all payments."

I had given attorney Shapiro proof that the money for the house's down payment was in my own account prior to the marriage. Proof that for every $100 Haywood deposited into our checking account, I deposited five or six hundred. (I proved this by taping together the checks that I retrieved from the trash.) Proof that 90% of our home was modestly but nicely furnished and belonged to me prior to the marriage, and the other 10% was purchased in my name. Proof that bonds were taken out of his monthly check in his mother's name. Proof that he made occasional deposits into a bank account in LaGrange. And proof how all of his family benefited from the many cars he purchased.

I never received a notice again. It was a struggle for Haywood, but he paid for the car. His health began to fail, and he retired from his job early. Soon he had two brain surgeries. Since we were getting a divorce and he was no longer at home, I was not given the details of his surgery. At this writing, I am told he is in a private nursing home, being cared for by a niece.

After the hearing I called Auntie Olivia, who said, "I am very happy everything turned out well for you. Now I can die in peace. Angeline wanted me to go to sleep. I told her I was waiting for your call. Tell me everything that happened today."

I told her everything, including Haywood's offer after the hearing to give me a ride home, an offer that I declined. I told her I remembered what she said about the car. She said, "Never forget it. Renee, I have prayed for you every day. In the past you made your husband, your children, and your home your first priority. Now that the divorce is behind you, save a few pennies when you can. Put Renee first for a change, travel when you can, and enjoy your life. Keep these words I say close to your heart, Renee:

Weeping may endure for a night,
but joy cometh in the morning.

Psalm 30:5

"Let God be your hiding place. Keep your hands in His hands, and all will be well with you. God did not give me a child. But if he had given me a daughter, I would want her to be just like you. I love you, little girl. I can close my eyes now."

At midnight, the phone rang. It was Angeline: "I call with bad news. Olivia died two hours after speaking to you on the phone. She knew she was dying and said she would be ready to go to sleep once she talked with you. Olivia made all of her own funeral arrangements and left an envelope with me for you. It is your plane fare so you can attend her funeral. Get your ticket; the money will be here for you when you arrive. My daughter will pick you up at the airport."

When I arrived, Angeline gave me a small manila envelope. The writing appeared to be that of Auntie Olivia's. My name was written on the front, and on the back flap was written "$3000." The envelope contained $500.

Aunt Olivia's love for me was genuine. She could not have loved me more if I were her own child. She wore her garments well—garments of an angel.

Chapter 10

I was buying my gas and having my oil changed at a service station two blocks from the hospital. One day Haywood stopped there and cursed out the attendant. After that, I was afraid to trust them under the hood of my car and started getting service at another station along the way. One morning in 1985 I was reading a magazine, waiting for my car to be finished, when a man walked in and called my name. I looked up into Felton's face. He was as surprised to see me as I was to see him.

He asked, "How did you happen to stop here?" I said, "I have been getting gas and oil changes here for quite awhile." "That is impossible," he replied, "I would have seen you. This is my place."

I was shocked. There were four stations in a three-block area, and that was where I had stopped. The last time I had spoken to Felton, he was located elsewhere. The attendant said, "She has been coming here for a long time and always comes around 8 AM." That was why Felton hadn't seen me: he never went in to work until 11 AM.

Felton then surprised me with his next comment: "You did not marry the man that gave you those beautiful rings all those years ago. Three years later, you married a different person. You went back to school and are a nurse now. You had several of Beverly's children for a while, and now your Korean daughter-in-law lives with you. Also, you have been divorced now for almost a year."

I could not believe this and asked, "How did you know?"

"While visiting a very close friend who lives in Rockford, Illinois, she asked why I had not remarried. I told her I had met the love of my life but had failed to take advantage of the opportunity to marry her. My friend was curious, so I told her about you. I also told her about your family and mentioned your brother Carlton's name. We discovered that she and your brother's wife were good friends. Whenever I wanted to know how you were doing, I would call my friend and ask, "How is the love of my life?" We would laugh, and the next day she would call your sister-in-law. So for thirteen years I kept up with you." After that, Felton and I started talking on the phone again.

In 1987, Dietra and I went on vacation to Canada with a group of her coworkers. The day after we returned, she and I stopped by Felton's place to show him our photos. Felton and I started dating after that.

The next day, Dietra's daughter called to tell me that her mother had been rushed to the hospital. When I arrived, the doctor told me that Dietra had suffered a stroke. I thought about the blazing heat we had just experienced in South Dakota as we returned from our trip. The bus had broken down, and we had to stand outside in the sun, since the repair shop's owner said that there were too many of us to fit inside.

My brothers and I were concerned about Dietra. Since I was no longer married but they were, we decided that Dietra and I would sell our three-bedroom homes and buy a building together.

Dad and his wife Mattie were not well. They lived east on 93rd. Dietra, recuperating from her stroke, lived west on 107th, and there I was, west on 78th. It was not easy for me to be running all over. I believed that Dad was going to outlive his wife, and it would be easier if we were all in one place. So Dietra and I purchased a three flat on West 79th Street.

❧

As I unpacked boxes, hung paintings, and put linen in place, I thought of all the people I had shared my home with. There was Eva, whose mom had put her out of the house. I admired her desire to stay in school. Not only did she finish high school, but she met her future husband while with my family and married out of my house. I also remembered Uncle Paul, whom I loved him dearly. A godly man, he was special to us; he and his family lived with us for about five months.

I listened to my music and thought that this would be a different experience, the very first time I would live alone (although Dietra lived upstairs). My son Gamal had finished a course in Orthopedics and was working as an Ortho tech at Cook County. He, Soon-Na, and their three daughters had bought a home on West Francisco. My other son Gregory was also living on his own.

In June, Felton started telling me he wanted to be with me. He said, "I had an opportunity to marry you once; I do not want to lose you again." Seven years had passed since Haywood and I had divorced, and I had started praying for a companion. Since I knew something about Felton, I had no fears.

Sometimes when Felton had a long drive to pick up parts for a car, he would call. If I was awake, I'd ride with him. We would go out for dinner, and since he knew of my love for music, he'd get us tickets to musicals. So we got to know each other again.

He'd also clip cartoons about love and mail them to me. One Valentine's Day he called and said, "I want you to read every line on page 107 of the *Chicago Sun-Times*." There I found an ad telling me he loved me. In September he gave me an engagement ring, and in November we were married.

Mattie, Dad's wife, died in December. Since Dad's health was not the best, I brought him to live with Felton and me. This was no surprise to Felton, since prior to our marriage I had told him this would happen.

Dad was to have home care. I did not want strangers coming into my home and was told I could get a relative to come in and assist with Dad's care. It would be done through the home care agency. Soon-Na, Gamal's wife, signed up for the job. The agency said she had to pass a test. Since she did not read English well, the agency allowed her to have the questions read to her so she could answer "true" or "false." She passed the exam.

I was shocked to learn that Dad had no insurance of value. I told my siblings that his meager Social Security allowance would have to be set aside for future burial purposes. They all agreed. Dad was given a monthly allowance.

In 1992, Felton's brother Hilliard came to visit. The three of us drove to Kansas to visit their stepfather. While driving, the two brothers disagreed on something, and Felton became angry. Later in private I told him he was wrong. He became even angrier and said that right or wrong, I was supposed to agree with him.

When we returned home, Felton made my dad an issue. He said I was doing too much for my father and that he should live with my siblings sometimes. I had to tell Felton, "All of your needs are being met, and I am not neglecting you. I will not let you dictate to me what I can or cannot do for my dad. I love my father. I told you that before we were married." He resented my dad's presence, but never said anything again.

He later began to complain about Gregory and my grandchildren. I told him, "I am aware of all the things you do for your son and his family. Please do not upset me by complaining about what I do for mine." Felton could not understand the closeness my children and I shared. I told him he should work at developing a closer relationship with his sons. Whenever we had a family gathering, I would always ask his sons to come.

When I would go on a trip, Dad would stay with my brother Robbie and his family until I returned. In 1993, Dietra and I were planning to visit an aunt in New York. Our tickets were already purchased, but Dad then broke his hip and Felton had to have major surgery. Although they were both home and recuperating, I gave my ticket to my niece and stayed home with Dad and Felton.

Robbie was at the station every day taking care of Felton's business. My brother, being a man of great integrity, significantly increased the day's receipts. The business was handled in such a way that it cut down on some of the stealing and there were more frequent drops to the safe.

I regretted not going to New York. People did not expect me to be home, so the calls from the women came.

As I was preparing to take Felton to the doctor one morning, the phone rang. Felton assumed I would be on the phone a long time, so he went to the bedroom and made a call himself. He lay flat on his back with his feet on the floor and looked up at the ceiling. He was so into his conversation that he did not notice when I entered the room. After a few seconds, he realized I was there and hung up the phone without ending his sentence. He had a strange look on his face; it was obvious he had been talking to a woman. I said, "I am ready when you are ready," nothing more.

When we returned from the doctor's office, I told Felton I did not care who he talked to, but I did not want women calling the house or him calling them from the house. The conversation was not about business. He said, "I was not talking to a woman." I looked at him and just shook my head. He then changed his story and admitted, "Yes, it was a woman—my cousin."

Felton completely ignored my request. Many nights before I could get to work, he would be on the phone talking to this one lady. My dad would be lying in the bedroom, listening. Dad never said anything, but I watched the relationship between he and Felton go from warm and friendly to very formal.

Felton's recuperation went well, and he was soon back to work. My brother continued to open up the station every morning and assist him. Felton always left for work around 11 AM and rarely came home before 10 PM. After working all night, I would be up by 1 PM and would have dinner ready by 4 PM. I would feed Dad, then drive twenty minutes to the station to take Felton a hot meal.

My husband's behavior was obviously no better at the station than at home. I arrived one evening with his dinner when my brother told me, "Renee, you need to get your rest; if you do not take care of yourself, no one else will." He did not have to say anything else; I got the message. I never said one word to him about Felton's behavior. I was too ashamed.

Willis, one of Felton's employees, looked up to Felton as a father figure and was disturbed with his behavior. Willis gave me all the respect a son could give to a mother. He was always telling customers what a beautiful person he thought I was. It was difficult for him to see that Felton's behavior with women did not change after we were married.

On one occasion, Willis got so drunk after witnessing some of Felton's behavior that he could not function on the job. My brother called me to say he did not know what was wrong with Willis and asked if I could come talk to him. When I came, Willis broke down and cried. At first he said he did not wish to talk. I replied, "When you went to take Felton the checks this morning, you found a woman there, and it bothered you." "How did you know that?" he replied. I did not know; he had just told me with his response.

It turned out that the lady Felton most often talked to thought I was his live-in girlfriend. So when the lady called the next time, I answered the phone and told her, "I am Mrs. Howard, Felton's *wife*."

She said, "I have known Felton for twenty years; he is not married." Since she did not believe me, she told Mark, one of the attendants at the station, "Felton's girlfriend says she is his wife." He replied, "If you are talking about Renee, she *is* his wife."

She then confronted Felton: "Both Mark and Renee say she is your wife." He responded, "Who are you going to believe—me or them?" Of course, she chose to believe him, and the calling continued.

It was very painful for me for Felton to imply that I was lying when I said I was his wife. It was at that point the very bottom dropped out of our marriage. The love I felt for him slowly drained away.

I told Felton that if he did not stop the phone calls, I would. I knew how. I insisted he tell the lady I was his wife. He refused, saying, "I have never told her that you were not my wife." "That is not the problem," I replied, "The problem is you never told her I was."

He still refused, so I gave him a choice. I told him I would never mention her name again, but if she called our house or if he called her from our house, then I would call her. Felton insisted that he had never given the lady our phone number, but our unlisted phone number automatically showed up on her caller ID. I continued, "I do not care how many women you talk to. They are your living. You have as many women customers as you do men, if not more. But I know who this lady is, where she lives, and that she is married, among other things."

He did not believe me. The calling continued. While we were having breakfast one morning, I reached for the phone, unannounced, and dialed the lady's home. When her husband answered the phone, I said, "Hello! I am Renee, the wife of Felton. I would like for him to speak to your wife." Felton, who sat speechless, refused to take the phone. I then told Felton, "I did not ask you to stop seeing or calling her. I only asked for respect here in our home. That it not be done from here." "You are crazy!" he exclaimed, to which I responded, "No, I am not crazy. There is a phone across the street; you can do your calling from there."

Need I say there was never another phone call?

In 1995, the big toe on Felton's right foot became gangrenous and had to be amputated. I continued to care for both Dad and Felton and prayed constantly that God would keep Dad on his feet until I could retire. I did not want Dad to want water and have to wait for Felton to give it to him.

Chapter 11

I t was 1996, and I was happy. Dad was alert, still on his feet, and attending church every Sunday. I had finally reached age 65 and was looking forward to retiring. I wrote a retirement statement for my supervisor. The Nursing Director was impressed with my statement and asked if it could be published in the hospital newspaper. It appeared in the April 1996 *Tablet* and read, in part:

U. of C. Medical Center
Renee C. Howard Retires!

In June of 1948 when I graduated from high school, the class prophecy stated that in 20 years I would be employed at the University of Chicago. In February of 1968, almost exactly 20 years later, I was hired at the hospital as a nurse's aide.

When my mother died, I was 10 years old and was told that angels would take care of her. From that day on, I believed that angels would take care of me, also. I firmly believe that at strategic times God put in place real, live angels to touch my life. I met some of them at the hospitals.

Madelyn Spragle, RN, was there to touch my life. Not only did she encourage me to return to school, she provided me with an expensive book... Shortly after I finished, pharmacist E.D. Miller and RN Beola Semious, along with Armenta Kelly...urged me to go back to school again. Their concern...made the difference. I went back to school and became an RN.

There was Carol Reliford, a natural born teacher. When fetal monitoring came to the third floor, five of us had great difficulty. On her own time in her home, she tutored us and made fetal monitoring seem like the ABCs. Betty Zeisler, night supervisor...showed concern for everyone. Then there was Elsie Shiohara; she was truly an angel. She trained me to fill in for both herself and Ms Zeisler. I knew that she wanted me to be my best. Sadie Smith was another angel in my path. We attended school together in 1968 and were supportive to each other as coworkers...

When I think of where I was when I came to the hospitals and where I am as I leave, I know that I have been blessed. If I could have one wish come true, it would be that as employees enter this great institution, they would leave their personal biases and prejudices outside and resolve to be a positive force in the life of at least one human being. Then we could say not only can one find medicine and nursing at the forefront in the hospitals but with humanity as well.

Renee C. Howard, RN

✆

A few weeks before my last day at work, I stopped by the station to see my brother Robbie and told him I was thinking about writing a book. I thought it would be good to write about the struggles of a single mom, since I had been one most of my life.

"Do you have a title?"

"Yes. *Garments of Angels*."

"If that is your dream, you will have to do more than just talk about it. I remember hearing you say this a year ago. You need pen and pad in hand, if it is going to become a reality."

"Yes," I answered, "I will start now that I am retiring."

~

Since retiring causes one to reminisce, I thought about the past. My maternal grandfather, Robert, was a farmer and a minister. We were raised close to the church. Now my brothers Carlton, Robbie, and Elliot were all ordained ministers. Roland was not an ordained minister but a minister at heart—his life centered on the church and its care.

My dad was a barber most of his adult life, owning his own shop most of those years. Dad took great pride in the fact that Dietra, Bette, and I were RNs. He marveled at the fact that Gamal had taken a course in orthopedic technology and today is an orthopedic instructor. Gamal was always telling Dad he was going to invent a splint, and Dad would always say, "Don't tell me about it. Show it to me."

Gamal encouraged two of his daughters, Lucinda and Lisa, and two of his nephews, Edmond Jr. and Michael, into becoming Ortho Techs. Also, Dad felt it was an apparently inherited DNA trait stemming from his great-grandfather, Dr. Edwin C. Dancy.

Now, years later, here I was, using my skills to care for Dad.

~

February came, and I stood in the window and looked out at the snow. Finally I did not have to get out of my warm bed at 10 PM to go out into the frigid weather. Boy, was I happy.

I began to enjoy my retirement and started watching the Oprah show. Now I had the time to curl up with Oprah's book of the month.

March 7th came, and another big snow. Dad and I sat up watching TV until 1 AM. Around 5 AM, I got up, went to the front window, and looked at the snow. Then I checked on Dad. He lay there very still, pale. I looked to see if his chest rose and fell. It did not. Then I reached to feel the carotid pulse. There was none. No air came out of his nostrils. God had answered my prayers. I had prayed many times for Dad to stay on his feet until I came home for good. After I was retired only six weeks, Dad was gone.

I called my siblings so we could make arrangements. They said whatever I decided would be fine, since I had taken care of Dad. His money paid for everything. No one argued; everything was peaceful.

After I paid all Dad's medical bills, there was $1000 left. We decided we would visit our stepmother, Mama Eria. Three carloads went to see her one weekend, everything paid for with Dad's money.

ᴄᴦ

My daughter Bev came to help with a family reunion; I had not seen her since Christmas. I could tell she was not well, so I insisted she see a doctor as soon as the festivities were over.

I thought she had pneumonia, but she was had lung cancer. When she showed me her medicines, I knew doctors did not expect her to live long.

Three days a week I took her to the hospital for her treatment. I tried to get her to come live with me; however, she preferred to stay home. On November 21st I received a phone call from my granddaughter telling me to come: her mom was dead.

There I was, eight months after Dad's death, making arrangements for my own daughter's funeral.

Chapter 12

The year 1996 was finally coming to an end. It had not been an easy year for me. God had answered my prayers concerning my dad, who had lived a good life and was 84 years old when he died. However, I was at times despondent thinking about Bev's death.

There was little or no communication between Felton and me. I lost myself in music and reading.

I wrote to Oprah Winfrey, asking for tickets to attend one of her shows. I stated I was writing a book. Of course there were only a few pages; it was all mostly in my head. I did not realize then how much was involved in publishing a book.

Some time later, I received a call from the show, telling me I had seats for two. I was deliriously happy. You would think I had just received an invitation to Buckingham Palace. Felton was equally happy.

On the day we attended the show, there was a big snow. I was thankful I had Felton to take me. That day we were all given Wally Lamb's book *She's Come Undone*. It was a great day for both Felton and me; I was happy for weeks thinking about it. Attending the show gave us something to talk about.

✎

The following spring, Bette said, "Mom, you need to get away. In June I will be going on a business trip to New Orleans. It would be good for you to go. It would give you an opportunity to see Edmond."

So in June, Bette and I arrived in New Orleans. Edmond met us at the airport with a map in hand; we were on our way to check into our rooms at the Brent House at the Oschner Foundation Hospital. The enclosed area between the two buildings was ornamented with exotic flowers, trees and a self-playing piano. Its soft, classical music made it a nice place to sit and relax.

Bette then asked, "Mom did you bring a writing pad?"

"No," I replied.

"In the morning, stop in the gift shop and get one. It is peaceful and quiet here, so this is a good time for you to start working on that book you are always saying you are going to write."

The following morning I had breakfast, then went to the gift shop and purchased a writing pad.

The next morning, after showering and ordering breakfast, I opened the curtains and beheld the beauty below. The tenth floor was just high enough to enjoy the view and thank God for my eyesight.

The green trees and grassy slopes were beautiful to behold. I stood and looked out at New Orleans with its tall buildings and the Superdome. To my left I cold see the rippling waves of Lake Pontchartrain with numerous boats sailing in its waters. The fast moving waves let me know the lake was very much alive. When I looked to my right down Causeway Blvd., I could see the great Huey P. Long Bridge.

There was a knock at the door: breakfast had arrived. I sat at the window with the beautiful view, in awe of what was before me. Listening to my music, I began to write, and before I knew it, it was 2 PM. Out across most of the city's hazy sky, I could see repeated streaks of lightning, but down Causeway Blvd., the sun shone bright with no sign of rain.

I stood looking at the vast skyline before me with thoughts of pride for my daughter, Bette, who was raised in a single parent home by a mother on public assistance. Often we did not know where the next meal would come from, but she now sat in corporate meetings making decisions that would affect many people. I appreciated the fact that she realized it was not her knowledge alone, but God had given her favor.

Chapter 13

After retirement I thought I would volunteer at one of the local hospitals. However, Dietra decided to become a foster parent and convinced me to do the same. We applied for a license and began fostering in 1998.

I asked for one child—a girl age four through eight. But to keep a family of children together, we each took two children. Dietra took the youngest and the oldest—two girls. I took the middle two—Teresa, age six, and Ted, age ten.

When the agency called to say that the children would be arriving soon, Dietra's youngest daughter stopped in to see me. She said, "Renee, the children that come into your home are going to really be blessed. You are such a loving person. You have so much to give." It made me feel good to hear her say that. It was the nicest thing she ever said to me.

The children and I were a blessing to each other. It was a reciprocal affair: I showered them with love, and they loved in return. They brought back laughter and life into our home. In their own way they let me know that I was an important factor in their lives.

I gave the children an option. They were told they could call me Ms. Howard, Ms. Renee, or Auntie Renee. They chose to call me Auntie Renee. I carried the children with me everywhere I went: to church, to shop, and to visit. If an invitation was extended to me and the children were not welcome, I did not go.

I treated the children as though they were my own. In fact, everyone thought they were my grandchildren, since they looked so much like my own. Teresa reminded me of my daughter, Bev.

Once a month we attended a parent meeting at the center. The social workers often voiced their opinions on how happy the children were. You could tell they were receiving A-one care. The children's lawyer also marveled over the placement.

Teresa was almost seven and had not yet attended school, but she left my home an A student. Her teacher was surprised to learn she was a foster child and said she thought Teresa was my grandchild. Early on I told the social worker I would consider becoming Teresa's legal guardian, if she was not reunited with her mother.

Ted, the 10-year old, was a sweet and loving child, but in his mind he was a man. For so long he had taken on the role of protector for his three siblings that he felt older. In fact, he said to me many times, "I am the man." I told Ted he was a child, and I expected him to perform like a child.

I kept Ted about eight months. Almost every morning before school, he would challenge my authority. My husband and I had misunderstandings, but there was no toe-to-toe arguing. Not so with Ted; at least two or three times a week, it was almost word-for-word.

I began to document Ted's behavior for the social worker. I told Ted there were 30 lines on the paper and if he caused me to document all the way down to the 25th line, I would have to consider giving him up.

Someone told the children there was a way they could go live with a friend of their mother's, which would allow them to see their mom whenever they liked. So Ted and his oldest sister got together and said I struck Teresa, hoping this would let them move.

The social worker and director came. Of course, the children admitted they were not telling the truth. But I became concerned about what this would do to my reputation, since this was considered child abuse and had to be documented. I was both hurt and angry, because I knew an adult had influenced the children.

Ted told the worker he did not have any privacy because I looked through his chest drawers. I washed, ironed and kept his clothing folded in the drawers, so naturally I looked in them. He was told by the agency he could have a shoebox, and I would not be allowed to look in it.

I told the agency I paid my mortgage and made the rules for my home. A shoebox could hold drugs, a gun, or any number of things. If they insisted that Ted have such a box, they would have to remove him.

The people at the agency had great respect for me but were not exactly crazy about me. I had challenged them before on behalf of the benefits due the children. Now they pleaded with me to give Ted another chance. I said I would.

But the morning challenges with him continued. On December 8, Ted pushed my button to the limit. I called his worker and told her my blood pressure would not allow me to keep him any longer.

When she came for him, he tried to be a man by not crying. It was very difficult for him when he learned he would be leaving and his sister would remain. Once outside, he fell upon the worker's car, crying and pleading to make me let him stay. It was heartbreaking for all of us.

My sister Dietra said it was going to be very hard for Ted, since he was going into a home that had three or four other boys. She told me, "His snow white tee shirts and socks are going into the wash with the others, and that is were the fighting is going to start. You kept his clothes too neat and orderly."

Dietra was right. We soon learned Ted was having problems, and he complained that the other boys wanted to wear his clothing and the foster mother saw nothing wrong with it. Two months after leaving my home, Ted exploded and cursed out everyone in the home. I was surprised, because no one ever heard him use profanity during the eight months he lived with me.

Ted was assigned a mentor. After he was moved a second time and failed to make it, his mentor took him in. But Ted eventually became an A student.

Since we had sleeping space for two children, the agency immediately asked me to take in another little girl. Terri was five years old and ready for kindergarten. I told Teresa and Terri that although they were not blood sisters, they were Christian sisters while in my home, and that was how I expected them to behave. Teresa immediately took on the posture of being the big sister by giving orders, while Terri would remind her she was not the boss. The two of them got along well, and the three of us went everywhere together. Lisa and Lavette, Gamal's daughters, were very helpful, taking care of the girls' hair for me.

Felton was initially receptive to being a foster parent, realizing it brought life back into our home. However, in time he showed signs of quiet resentment, although he was never mean to the children. When I would prepare to do something with or for the children, he would insist I do something for him first. I would always comply with his wish. Felton thought I loved the children more than I did him. Except for being intimate, I knew my duties as a wife and carried them out to perfection. But I felt no desire for a man—not for him or anyone else. He had caused me to lose those feelings. I felt drained.

Many times when I was asking God to give me a companion, I should have just asked God to fill my life. The children did that for me; we were good for each other.

✆

Felton was a noncompliant diabetic and had other health issues. He did not follow the doctor's instructions and would become angry when I reminded him. Although he was told to wear special shoes, he refused, since they were not attractive. He would wear generic sneakers and would become belligerent if I told him they were not good for his feet.

In time the toe area flared up again, becoming gangrenous. After many weekly trips to doctors over a period of six months, it was decided the leg would have to be amputated. Felton settled for his original physician and was scheduled for surgery during the last week of August 2000.

I was scheduled to attend a workshop in Anderson, Indiana, the second week of July. I would be gone one week, and Felton's cousin and son were to take care of his feet in my absence. Teresa and Terri would stay with Soon-Na and the girls. When I returned, however, Felton was unhappy with the care he received from his cousins, who did not always come. I was scheduled to attend a family reunion in Philadelphia the last weekend in July, but Felton and his family did not think I should go.

I spoke to his physician, who said, "By all means, go! You will have your hands full after his surgery. It will be a while before you will get a vacation. Go! Go!"

I made arrangements for Lucinda and Lisa, my granddaughters who were Ortho Techs, to care for Felton's feet while I was away. Every evening, my son Gamal would drop them off at my house to care for Felton and he would return to pick them up.

Felton was pleased with the girls' work and told them I would pay them when I returned. When I came back, I asked the girls, "How did things go?" They replied, "Granddaddy said you would pay us when you got home. But we do not want to be paid, Granny. We took care of him because he's your husband and we love you."

When Felton went into the hospital, his doctor repeatedly said he was afraid to put Felton to sleep, because he might not awaken. We had been aware of this for some time. However, Felton survived the surgery.

A week later he required additional surgery; prior to this surgery, he suffered a massive stroke. He was in Intensive Care and paralyzed from the waist down. After his tubes were removed, Carlton, Robbie, and I sat at Felton's bedside.

Felton looked at me and said, "Di-di-di-did I te-te-tell you-you-you today th-th-that I love you?"

With unbelief in his voice, my brother asked, "What did he say?"

"He said, 'Did I tell you today that I love you?'"

"I thought that was what he said," Robbie replied.

I did not say anything. I was equally shocked to hear his words. But I ran my hand across Felton's brow and my fingers through his hair. During the early days of our marriage, Felton loved for me to run my fingers gently through his hair and massage his scalp. It was always done as an act of affection.

A doctor came into the room. When Felton spoke to me, the doctor asked what he had said. I told him Felton had said, "Introduce my doctor to my Pastor." He was referring to Robbie.

"You understand everything he says?" the doctor asked.

"Yes. But he has suffered a stroke."

The doctor disagreed, but I did not debate him. The next day when I arrived, they said Felton had indeed suffered a stroke. Since he had also contracted pneumonia and had to be intubated, Felton's primary physician and I discussed whether or not Felton should be resuscitated, if necessary.

I started looking for Felton's necessary papers and discovered they were missing from the house. While I was at my family reunion, those papers had been removed. I knew Felton had made out a will, because I was present when it was done and was knowledgeable of its contents. I do not believe anyone took undue liberties in my home in my absence. The papers were not there because Felton had removed them or given them to someone. I fully believe that whatever the reason, God was in the plan. I believe that everything God wants me to have, I will receive.

The doctors were finally able to get Felton's temperature down. He tubes were removed again, and he breathed on his own. But at times he appeared to be semi-comatose. The doctor asked if Felton had told me prior to our marriage that he knew he would one day be an amputee. I told the doctor Felton had not. According to the doctor, two years prior to our marriage, Felton was told that would happen.

After four weeks in the hospital, Felton was ready to be discharged and would need around-the-clock care. I was making preparations to get him into a nursing rehab center only five minutes from our house. I could be there for him every day. But his family was not pleased. One relative said to me, "You mean you are going to put him in a nursing home?" "Yes," I replied, "Those are my plans. I cannot possibly stay awake for 24 hours. Right now he needs around-the-clock care."

I was to finalize the paperwork on the Tuesday after Labor Day. But at 3 AM on Monday morning, the hospital called to say that Felton had expired. He lived a week longer than I thought he would; my nursing experience told me it would have taken a miracle. It was his plan that I would be there to care for him once he became an amputee. That was not to be. I believe those were not God's plans for me.

Felton had three insurance policies, and his beneficiaries were his son by his first marriage as well as a grandson. I did not have a problem with that, since I, too, had good insurance that named my children as beneficiaries. However, I had a problem with his family wanting me to pay for the funeral.

I made it plain that the person whose name was on the insurance policies should and would have to bear that expense. I knew enough that the sum total was more, more, more than enough to pay for a funeral.

Felton's only brother flew in for the funeral. He stayed with me and made it clear he understood what I was going through.

But one of Felton's former employees called another former employee and said, "Man, what is this I hear? Renee refused to bury Felton?" His friend replied, "I am glad she had that much sense! Renee is a good person. I have known her almost as long as I've known him. She took good care of him. You did not get the whole story. Felton had three policies, but her name was not on one of them. Would you not think if you left someone's name on your insurance that the first thing they would do is see that you were buried?" The first employee responded, "Man, you have got to be joking. That is not the way it was told to me. I am glad she had that much sense. You know, Renee is such a quiet person. I have to agree she took good care of him. Waited on him hand and feet."

At the funeral, only four or five of Felton's family members spoke to me. As far as the others were concerned, I was not there. I thank God for giving me a loving family and a church family that were there for me. My family showed their love and gave me support. My church family officiated and served the repast, which they paid for.

I planned the entire service. One of Felton's relatives who had played for many funerals said, "The service was very dignified and had class. You did a beautiful job." She was one of the few who spoke to me that day.

Chapter 14

When Felton had his first surgery, he had received an offer to buy his station. I had told him he should sell while he had an offer, because he would never work again. He did not listen to me and began to get further and further behind with his taxes.

Two years prior to his death, he rented the station to a young man name José. José was always late on his rent, sometimes by several months. I told José that things would be different now that he had to deal with me. He had let the place get in horrible condition, and the neighbors were complaining. José also had another station that he kept in immaculate condition. After I'd given him his third eviction notice, he knew I meant business: I was not going to be a pushover. He moved, put a padlock on the door, and never said a word.

One day Dietra happened to pass by the station and told me it appeared to be empty. I went to check. She was right. I called Jose's home numerous times and never got a return call. José was not aware I knew the location of his second station, but I went there and spoke to a young man who promised to give me keys the next day.

A close friend of Felton's advised me to sell the station as soon as possible, or it would be lost to taxes. "It would be in your best interest, Renee," he said and then gave me the name of an agent. When I called the agent, he went with me to José's. We were given keys, but they did not unlock the iron gates or the locks on the door. So I called in a locksmith and had the locks removed and new ones installed.

After several months, we were able to get a buyer, although we had to sell the place for much less than its value. The overdue tax consumed almost half of the selling price. But I was so thankful to be rid of the headache. It was draining my energy.

∾

Teresa and Terri were good for me during that time. They were both scheduled to reunite with their mothers. I kept Teresa until school was out. I had become very attached to her; she was such a loving child. Getting her things together was difficult for me. She did not want to take everything, because she wanted to return every weekend to be with Terri and me and so she could go to church.

Lucinda, Lisa and Lavette were there to say good-bye. When the van pulled away with Teresa, Terri cried, "Thank you Jesus! Now I can be the big sister. When are you going to get another little girl, Auntie Renee?" My granddaughters and I thought we would never stop laughing.

Terri stayed with me for another year until school was out. Together Dietra and I fostered seven children. They were all reunited with their mothers, but I am told that at this time they are all back in the system. I pray for their safety and well-being.

In April, we decided to sell our home. Had I remained on West 79ᵗʰ, I am sure my doors would still be open to someone's child.

In September, we put our home on the market on a Wednesday. By the following Tuesday we had showed the place seven times and had six contracts. God was truly good. We were excited.

Just thinking about being closer to our church was making me happy. I would be able to attend Bible class and would have lots of time to practice my music lessons. I had bought and given away at least five keyboards in the past, since I wanted to instill music in some child in hopes that one day they would be a musician. The church purchased my beautiful console organ, and I replaced it with a smaller spinet.

I informed our tenant, a minister, that we were selling and recommended to the new owner that he keep her as a tenant. She came upstairs before I left and asked to pray with me. She then said, "Ms. Howard, you have been a blessing and an inspiration to me. I am going to miss you. Your children were wise to insist you give up this place. You are going to experience peace and happiness in your new home. You will have time to write. Your latter years will be your best."

Chapter 15

Fifteen days before Christmas, I was finally moved into my new home in a senior village. From day one I was very excited about moving into "The Rose Gardens." Watching the trees and shrubbery blossom and change hues added to the excitement. It was wonderfully serene to sit at the dining table and watch a bluebird, cardinal, or some other bird play in the quiet garden. When I watched the trees bud and burst open with blossoms of many bright colors, I thought of the awesomeness of God and all His goodness.

I looked forward to meeting the other seniors and sharing the retirement years. When I moved in, only eleven families lived in the community. Two weeks later, my sister Dietra moved into The Rose Gardens, too.

Everyone always knew when a new family came. So of course I knew about the man who had suffered a stroke and moved in five months later.

One warm afternoon I was standing on my patio, watering the plants. I looked up and saw this man walking on the other side of the street, pushing a pram. His gait was no more than a shuffle. I thought, "Oh my God, he will never make it back to his home!" I cut the water off, went across the street, and spoke to him:

"You are a long way from home. Are you sure you will be able to make it back?"

"Oh, yes. I am a great walker. My name is Peter. What is your name?"

"My name is Renee."

"Yes, yes. The man told me about you."

"What man? What man are you talking about?"

"The man by me."

"Do you mean Karl?"

"Yes, yes—Karl. He told me all about you."

Peter began to cry, waving his arms about and speaking in a very emotional voice: "You have a sister who lives here. You have a brother who is the pastor of a church."

"Yes, that is true."

"I am looking for the church! I am looking for the church!"

"Don't cry," I said, putting my arms around him, "Would you like to go to my church?"

"Yes, yes I would."

"I will take you to my church, if you like."

He stopped crying, gave me a long look, and then said, "You would do that for me?"

"Yes. When would you like to go?"

"To the next service!"

"That will be tomorrow. I will leave for Sunday school at 9:30, then come back for you at 11:30."

"No, no. I will leave at 9:30 with you! I am a widower. I lost my wife. It will be two years this September." He began crying again. This time his whole body was shaking, trembling. I again put my arms around him.

"Don't cry. It's going to be all right. I am a

widow. I too lost my husband. It will be two years this September. Believe me, it's going to be all right."

"God is with me," he said, raising his arms to the sky. "It is not by chance that you and I have met here. God is in the plan. You are an angel, Renee. God sent you to me. No, it is not by chance."

As I tried to comfort him, I saw several neighbors watching us from their doorways. I looked around to see who would help me pick him up from the ground if he should fall. He assured me that he would be able to walk the circle back to his unit. We agreed again on the time I would pick him up for service. I then went back to the patio and resumed watering the plants, watching him until he turned the bend and was out of sight.

It was later that I learned that as Peter neared his home, he met two ladies coming from the clubhouse—my sister Dietra and cousin Marion. He told them he had just met a lady named Renee. "She is an angel!" he exclaimed. When they told him who they were, he said, "Very good, then, I have met *three* angels!"

Chapter 16

On Sunday morning, Dietra, Marion, and I picked up Peter for church. Once we arrived, he was given a warm reception. After service, he was invited to have dinner in my home with my family and Robbie, the pastor of our church. Whenever I invited someone to visit my church for the first time, I would invite them to share dinner at my home; the pastor would join us, too. This gave the visitor an opportunity to visit with Pastor in a more relaxed setting. That was the beginning of numerous dinners Peter would share with my family and me.

The second week, Marion and I went to Anderson University to a leadership retreat, so Dietra took Peter to church. The third week, the three of us picked him up again. It was then we learned that Peter could drive and had a van. We were all surprised. He said he knew his way to the church and would drive himself from now on.

Shortly after I met Peter, he called to say his children were having a birthday dinner for him at the clubhouse. Something small, he said. He asked if Dietra, Diane, and I would come. Diane was the first person Peter met when he moved into the community.

Peter's daughter, his son Perry, Perry's wife, several grandchildren, and some of Perry's in-laws also came. Dietra and I were asked a number of questions, but I do not remember Diane being questioned. We sang "Happy Birthday," and I remember someone telling Peter's age. I thought they said he was 71, but I might have been mistaken. I thought he was older. Gray or white hair can be deceiving.

Reflecting on this party later, I thought the dinner was an excuse for the children to scrutinize the women that were taking their father to church and visiting him in his home. I am sure I would have done the same thing, had it been my father.

Later Peter invited Dietra, Marion, and me to dinner at his home. When we arrived, Marion washed dishes and I prepared the table as Dietra looked on. Peter made a delicious French dish and several other savory dishes from his native land, India. Peter's son Perry came, and I set a place for him. Perry only had a bowl of soup, and after he felt comfortable with us being in his father's home, he excused himself and left. Then there was lots of talking and laughter.

After dinner as Marion and I were cleaning up the kitchen, Peter said, "I have a great idea! We should buy a big house and all of us move in together. We could each have our own private bedroom and bath." We looked at each other, and the four of us let out a roar of laughter. We laughed and laughed and laughed.

Peter attended church each Sunday and immediately became part of its family. Whenever the pastor came to visit my sister and me, he also visited Peter. Sometimes he would even visit Peter first.

One evening, one of the ladies at church wanted to know what, if anything, I knew about Peter. I told her that I knew absolutely nothing about him, only that he was a nice person, my neighbor, and seemed to be very sincere. Peter asked many questions, but I did not; I wait and let people tell me what they want me to know. Sometimes you ask a lot of questions and get a lot of lies. When I told Peter that I was questioned about him, he asked, "And what did you tell her?"

"What is there for me to tell anyone, except the truth? As far as I know, you are a nice person, my neighbor, a widower, and the father of three children. Beyond that, you are a stranger. I do not know anything about you, so that is what I told her. I know you are friendly and like to ask people in for tea. However, do not do that with any of our church women young enough to be your daughters. It will be frowned upon. People who respect you will lose that respect."

"Are you serious?"

"Very much so."

"You know, I was told—"he began. But I didn't let him finish.

"I am sure you have been told many things about my people that are not true. I can only tell you what is valid in my circle of people."

Peter loved to pose for photos with the young ladies, and he prepared to tell me the nature of his conversation with one young lady. I stopped him and said, "You owe me no explanations. The nature of your conversation with anyone is not any of my business."

"I learn something each time we talk, Renee."

❧

Six or seven weeks into our friendship, Peter called and asked if I would come talk with him, since he needed my help. He explained his culture, that he had not experienced "dating," and that he was not sure how he should do it. He then talked about the loss of his wife and began to cry, saying how he longed to have a companion: "I am looking for a companion. I've watched you close, Renee. Your resources are many."

I told him I thought he needed a man's advice. Although I was married more than once, I was quite naïve. I said, "If you do not remember anything I say, remember this: don't go looking; just let it happen. God knows your desires and needs. When you meet the person he has for you, it will just happen."

"Your brother said the same thing," he answered.

"If Pastor told you that, and you say I am now saying it, then there must be some truth to it."

I was not aware that Peter and my brother Robbie had had such a conversation, since Robbie would never divulge his conversations with people.

"Don't select someone young enough to be your daughter. She will not really want you, only what you have or what she thinks you have. A woman in her fifties will be in the prime of her life. She will want to be wined and dined and taken to the best places. In time you will not be able to keep up with her. Select a woman in her sixties— someone closer to your own age, someone who will be tired when you are tired and sleepy when you are sleepy. You don't want to push yourself trying to keep up with someone, trying to prove you are younger than you are. You want someone who will love you for who you are just as you are. Nothing and no one is perfect, but you will have many more happy days as you continue to grow older."

I named all the single women in our church and community and then continued, "A companion means something different to different individuals. To some it is a very close or special friend, but they do not sleep together. To some people, it is the person with whom they sleep, and to others it is their wife or husband. You need to define what a companion means to you."

He said, "I will never marry again. I am going to India soon and would like to take a companion with me. I would like to have someone to travel with me."

"I do not know anyone who would leave the United States and go to India. Not now with so much unrest in the East," I replied.

The next week he asked me to accompany him to pick up his eyeglasses. He offered to drive, but I said I would. We were on the "companion" subject again, and I named several ladies I thought he should get to know.

"I don't need names," he answered, "I already know who I want."

I was in the middle of an intersection and did not hear all he said, but I heard enough to almost came to a dead stop. Once I got through the traffic light, I asked, "What did you say?" He would not repeat it.

∾

Once while visiting my home, Peter admired my curtains, as most people do. He called one day and asked if I would bring the catalog and help him select curtains for his own windows. Marion, Dietra, and I went. We also carried a photo album. Peter had never been upstairs in the fellowship hall of our church, so I wanted him to see pictures of how nice it was. Peter's son Perry also came. When I told Perry I wanted his father to see the upper sanctuary, he said, "Dad can walk up those stairs." We were all surprised.

There were many pictures taken in the sanctuary, but Peter wanted to see every picture, even though there were at least two hundred. We came across a photo of me sitting outside church, wearing black and white plaid pants and a white sweater.

I asked, "Do you know this face?" "Yes," Peter replied, "I know it well. I see it in my sleep." I was not prepared for that answer, and just hurried and flipped the page. No one said anything.

Three or four weeks later, Peter and I were talking on the phone when Peter came right out and said, "I don't know how you feel about me, Renee, but you are my world. I am willing to give you unconditional love!"

I did not say anything; I did not know what to say. I just held the phone, since I hadn't expected that.

Loving a man, any man, was nowhere in my thoughts. I must say that the many overtures he made were very flattering, particularly since I believe that older men are not interested in women their own age. Even though Peter was now happy, I was aware that he came to our community a very lonely man.

❧

One of my most endearing moments with Peter was on a trip to a farmstand. On the way home, we stopped at Popeye's, a fast food place, and Peter told me I should order whatever I wanted. Our hands were very dirty from the farmstand, so I got a glass of water for our table. Taking Peter's hands in mine, I washed and dried them. His eyes never left my face.

Peter then took my hands in his and, with a tenderness I had never experienced, said, "I want to share something with you, Renee; you must never, never share it with anyone." I will never forget what he did. I looked at Peter and, as I always did, smiled and said nothing. After eating, we sat there an hour or more, talking and laughing.

❧

Peter wanted turnips. He was interested only in the bottoms, but I told him the tops were very good, too. So he decided he would cook the bottoms, I would cook the tops, and then we would share.

That evening I cooked the turnip tops, as well as fried corn, honey ginger carrots, cornbread muffins with broccoli, seasoned sliced tomatoes, cucumbers, and chilled melon for dessert. I prepared Peter's plate and then called to let him know I was coming shortly.

Peter said, as he always did, "The door will be open; just walk in." He then proceeded to tease me: "Renee, I believe you are in love; it is good to be in love." I listened but said nothing.

Arriving at Peter's, I placed some items on the counter and then said, "Do not tease me about being in love. I do not like that! I have no desire to be in love." He gave me a long look, shook his head slowly, and with a gentle but authoritative voice said, "It is not up to you. It is not up to you, Renee." He raised his fingers and beckoned for me to come. Like a robot I walked to him. Placing one arm around my shoulder, he looked me straight in my eyes and again said, "It is not up to you. Why do you feel that way, Renee?"

"There is nothing greater in life than to love and be loved in return. I do not believe there is a man out there that can give me the kind of unselfish love that I am capable of giving. So I choose not to love!"

Once more he said, "It is not up to you." Then he asked, "How many visas do I need, Renee?" I did not ask for clarification.

✣

Something happened to me that day. I was not the same. I did not understand my feelings, but I was very much aware of them. Sometimes I said to myself almost defiantly, "He doesn't know what he's talking about; it *is* up to me!"

After that, no longer did I open my door and walk out. Instead, I opened the door and looked out. If I saw Peter outside, I would not leave the house. Usually when the mailman came, several people would show up at the mailbox. Before I would join them, I would make myself wait to make sure that Peter was not there.

The same thing happened at church. If I saw him entering before he saw me, I would step inside the cloakroom until he entered the sanctuary. One Sunday, Dottie, the usher who stood outside the sanctuary doors with me, asked, "Why are you hiding from him?"

"I am not hiding," I countered.

"Yes you are! I've been watching you."

Needless to say, I stopped going into the cloakroom. Instead, I started standing with my back to the door, not looking at him until it was time for him to enter the sanctuary.

Chapter 17

Peter, Dietra, Lila, and Mary exercised in the clubhouse every weekday evening. I would not go. However, every evening I found myself at my living room window, waiting to see Peter walk across the street to the clubhouse. I would find myself at the window again when it was time for them to leave. I remember asking myself, "Why are you watching that man?"

On one of these occasions, I watched him get into his van, when all of a sudden it went into a tailspin, going around and around and around, like a spinning top!

I screamed, "Oh my God!" and was halfway to the car, when it came to a sudden stop. Peter waited awhile, backed up the van, and then drove it into the garage. By the time he got out of the van, I was standing inside the garage.

"Are you all right?" I asked. "What happened?"

"I'm all right, but I cannot talk about it now."

"God is taking care of you, Peter!" I exclaimed as I left.

Later Peter called and said, "I am fine, Renee, but I don't want to talk about that right now. Do you remember what you said to me when I got out of the van?"

"Yes."

"Say it again!"

"God is taking care of you."

"Those are very powerful words, Renee. I needed that. I will talk to you tomorrow."

✒

There were times when some of the women in the community would make negative remarks about Peter's condition. I would not engage in their conversations. It bothered me that someone would make belittling remarks about someone's physical condition. It was obvious they knew nothing of agape love. If I had been in Peter's condition, they would have said the same thing about me. But for the grace of God, it could be any one of us.

My eyes saw Peter's obvious handicap, but my heart, the seat of all emotions, saw only a kindhearted, sincere, quick-witted man who would have me laughing minutes after being in his company. We must remember in all our dealings with people that God is no respecter of persons and we should not be, either. God thinks no more of one of us than He does the other. In His sight we are all the same—His children.

✒

Peter called on Thursday and asked, "What are you doing, Renee?" I told him I was practicing my music lesson.

"You are hiding from me. I have not seen your face since Sunday."

"No, I am not hiding. I would never hide."

We talked for a short while. The following week, Peter called and asked again, "What are you doing?" After I told him, he replied, "You are hiding from me. I have not seen your face since Sunday. I want to see your face."

I assured him he would see me before Sunday. The next week he called and again asked, "What are you doing, Renee?"

"Thinking about you!" I said this time.

"How often do you think about me?" Peter asked, "Every day or every minute?"

"Both."

"What did you say?" he excitedly asked.

I spelled it out for him: "B-O-T-H!"

"Renee, you are in love! Can I now proclaim that Renee loves Peter?"

"Before I answer you, let me ask you a question."

"You can ask me anything."

"Can I now proclaim that Peter loves Renee?"

"Yes! Yes! You can tell the whole world!"

We talked and laughed for another ten or fifteen minutes.

❧

Shortly after that, Peter came to church in a very bad mood. He finally told us that he was arguing with some of his people from India. He said, "They are full of hate and know nothing of the love of God." Peter was always posing for photos with different young ladies and sent some of these pictures to India. We felt the confrontation was due to these photos.

In October, Peter told Dietra and Marion that his son Perry would be coming to church on Sunday. Instead, Peter's son Harold and his family came. They were warmly welcomed, as everyone usually is. At church, I could overhear Harold pointing me out to his wife, saying, "That's Renee, that's Renee." Both Harold and his wife seemed to really be into the message of the morning. Harold commented that it was a very nice church, and that since he himself was looking for a church home, he would not mind being there.

Two weeks later, Peter called, saying, "Please come, Renee. I need to talk to you about something dear to my heart. I need to know your thoughts."

When I arrived, he offered to make tea. We sat for a while, making small talk. Finally, with a somber look on his face, he said, "I will be leaving for India on the 19th of November." Then he said, "Look on the machine in the office and bring the paper there." I did and found the confirmation of his plane ticket. Then I sat, waiting to hear whatever was bothering him.

At last he asked, "What are your thoughts about a man going to another country and having sex there?"

I replied, "That is an individual decision that people make. Men and women do it all the time. Some people go abroad for just that reason. Me—I could never do that. Besides, it's a good way to pick up something that soap and water will not wash off."

"My family called a meeting," Peter explained. "I am to choose a companion in India." Hitting the table with his fist, he exclaimed, "I want to run away! I want to run away!" I listened and said nothing. Peter then asked, "What are your thoughts, Renee?" I looked at him a long time, straight in the face, before I answered:

"I know from experience that we tend to go looking for what we want, rather than being patient and waiting for God to send us what we need. I know, too, that it is not necessary for us to experience everything in life, when we can use wisdom and learn from the mistakes we see others make.

"Let me share something," I continued. "I had my chance 12 years ago. After seven lonely years, I asked God for a companion but did not wait for Him to send someone. Can you believe I thought He needed help from me? God, who is God all by Himself? He needed help from Renee?

"I did not wait for God to answer my prayers, and it turned out to be the biggest mistake of my life. One year after my marriage, it turned as sour as vinegar. The next two years were pure hell, and the next seven years, we lived a lie and were both miserable. We slept in the same bed, our feet and hands never touching.

"A close friend asked, 'How do you go through this?' And I said, 'I prayed to God for a companion and was too impatient to wait, so I am making the most of it. I took the vows; I am asking God to help me to be content. He gave me what I wanted. I did not wait for what I needed.'

"Peter, this is your season and your time; make the most of it. You say you never had the opportunity to be a bachelor. This is your time. Do the things a bachelor does. Date! But when it comes to choosing a permanent companion, choose wisely. Don't go looking; just let it happen."

There was no subject that Peter and I could not discuss. We talked a long time that evening about many things. Peter had a wit about him that made you feel relaxed in his presence.

"What about you, Renee?" he asked.

"I will be fine. You have given me something no other man has. I have that! There is nothing anyone can say or do that can take it away."

"Have I really?"

"Yes, you have!"

"What is that, Renee?"

"Everyone longs for unconditional love. No man has ever told me he was willing to love me unconditionally. You have done so more than once. Whether you meant it or not, the sincerity with which you said it causes me to smile inside, something I have not done in many years. This is your season, your time. I think you should go. Be happy. Use wisdom in your choice. I am sure your children worry about you living alone. They would worry less if someone were with you, and it would free them up to have more quality time with their families."

"If I should return with a companion, I would have to move," Peter responded. "I would not be able to live here."

"Why? Why not?" I asked.

He did not explain but just insisted he would have to move.

He looked at me for a long time and very quietly said, "You are special, Renee!"

❧

The light outside Peter's door had to be turned on and off manually. A week before he left, I purchased an automatic sensor light for him and promised I would bring it by after dinner. As usual, we greeted each other with the usual cheek-to-cheek show of affection that is so common among my family and church.

After laughing and talking for about an hour, I heard myself saying, "You know, the closer it gets for you to leave, I am experiencing an empty feeling. I am going to miss you." An indescribable fondness had grown between Peter and me.

"Do you really mean that, Renee?"

"You know I mean it."

An aura of peacefulness filled the room, and for a long time we just sat in silence. I do not have words to explain the feelings I had begun to feel for Peter. I do know it was a healing balm for all the pain I'd known from the past. I know that God knows better than I what is best for me. I thanked God for allowing our paths to cross. The rich, wholesome laughter erased the many disappointments from the past.

Peter, light bulb in his hand, shook his head slowly and with firm lips said, "This did it. I've thought about it for some time, and now I know it." He gave me a long hard look, and we continued our conversation.

When I stood to leave, I said, "There is no reason for a cheek-to-cheek goodbye. We did that when I came in, and I have not been here that long." I began walking toward the door.

Peter, following me, said, "I do not want a cheek-to-cheek from you today." With great emphasis he continued, "I want a *real* hug from you, Renee." Like a robot, I slowly turned to face him, my arms never leaving my side. It was a warm, gentle hug with an extra tightening of his arms—an affectionate, loving, tender hug. I stood there as though in shock. It seemed that all my energy left and was transferred to him. When Peter's arms released me, he said, "I want to share a passionate kiss with you before I leave."

"I do not share that kind of kiss with my friends," I replied.

"What did you say? Did you say you have never kissed a man?"

"No, I did not say that. I said, 'I do not share the kind of kiss you want with my friends.' A lot of me is invested in a kiss. I believe the kind of kiss you want is something very special. You only share that kind of kiss with one very special person in your life."

"I think you misunderstood me. There are two kinds of kisses."

"No, I understood you well. You said you wanted a very passionate kiss."

"Yes, I did say that, didn't I?"

"Yes, you did."

"You are so meticulous, Renee," Peter responded. Then with great deliberation, he repeated, "I want a very passionate kiss from you before I leave."

I looked at him and with equal deliberation, countered, "I will kiss you when you return, not before you go. When you return."

"Is that a promise?"

"It is a promise."

With that understanding, I left. Needless to say, I did not sleep well that night. I knew that Peter had deep feelings for me. Not only had he expressed himself verbally, but I could see it in his face, feel it whenever I was in his presence. Feel it in the tenderness with which he touched my hands. To have this at the beautiful age of 72 was healing for me.

But I thought it was important for me not to show my feelings. Men, especially elderly men, prefer younger women. Peter was no different from any other older man. Besides, he had already told me that his family had a meeting and he would probably return with a companion.

It did not make sense to share a passionate kiss with a man leaving in five days to select a companion. I felt safe making a promise because he would return with a companion, making a kiss totally inappropriate.

Chapter 18

The next morning when we spoke on the phone, Peter admitted, "I was very reluctant to ask you for a hug, Renee. I was so afraid you would say no. I think it was one-sided; I did all the hugging."

"Although my arms remained at my side, I assure you it was not one-sided. You did the giving; I did the receiving. I enjoyed the hug."

"Did you really, Renee?"

"Yes, I pushed the replay button many times."

"So did I."

We laughed and laughed.

Peter continued, "Tomorrow evening, please bring me the church email address and the pastor's phone number."

I called Peter the next evening, and he said, "Come; the door will be open." When I approached his home, I noticed that his window blinds were closed, a first since he had moved in. However, we had discussed the day before how he should leave his blinds when he left, so I thought nothing else of it.

Peter offered to make tea, and we talked about many things that evening. After about an hour of laughing and talking, he said, "Renee, I want you to spend a night with me—"

But I stopped him. "No, no, no; don't go there! You know I cannot do that. I cannot stand before the congregation serving communion with unclean hands."

He looked at me and said nothing. When I saw the rejected look on his face, I decided something and then added, "But I will kiss you before you leave."

"I would like that very much, Renee. I need to touch you!"

After a little while, I stood to leave. It was a very passionate kiss, ending with my head resting on his chest. With his right hand, the hand with the paralysis, Peter brought my face back to his. The second kiss was even more passionate than the first.

"We must stop!" I said, "We must not kiss again."

He held on to me as if his life depended on it. Finally he relaxed and left the room.

When he returned, holding his hands together, he said, "Renee, I am very happy with our friendship. I enjoy being with you. I wish we had spent more time together." As I walked to the door, he said, "When I return, I am going to London. Renee, I want to take you with me."

I said nothing and continued walking. When I reached the door, Peter deliberately repeated his statement: "When I return, I am going to London. I want to take you with me."

I did not respond but opened the door and walked out, not knowing that would be the last time I would see him.

The scent of him, the smell of him, was in my nostrils. It was a nice aroma that I could not shake for three days. In retrospect, I saw he had prepared for me. The soft smell of aftershave, the closed blinds. How naïve I was.

When we saw each other that last time, Peter spoke of his vulnerability while I sat and said nothing of my own. But I know that my vulnerability far exceeded his. To love is to be vulnerable; your feelings are out there, and they may not be handled with care.

✦

The following morning, Peter called.

"Good morning, Renee. How do you feel?"

"I feel good and bad," I replied.

"Me too, Renee. I feel nervous and shaky. I am weak, too weak to drive. I have never done anything irresponsible before in my life. Not after making a commitment. I want to run away."

I held the phone in silence, knowing he was struggling with his feelings.

"I am very weak, Renee."

"Yes, I know."

In a helpless voice, he continued, "I never dreamed I would come to this community and find love. Find someone who could love me. My children are in control of my very life."

I held the phone, making no response, so finally he said, "I guess that's how it is when you get old."

I still did not respond.

✦

After church on Sunday, Marion and my three granddaughters went to say goodbye to Peter. He asked the girls what they wanted him to bring them when he returned. They told him to bring whatever he chose. He said, "I will be writing to your grandmother. You are to tell her what you would like."

When they returned, Marion told me, "Renee, something is wrong with Peter. He does not look good. He has dark circles around his eyes as though he hasn't slept for days."

"Did he really?" I asked.

The girls replied, "Granny, he looked very tired."

I could not tell them I knew he was having some ambivalent feelings.

I called Peter on Monday to say goodbye and wish him well, but Peter wanted me to come on Tuesday to see him off. I wanted very much to look on his face one last time, but I knew it would be a painful moment for both of us. Since he cried so easily, I knew I would not be able to contain my own tears. So I chose not to go on Tuesday. If tears must come, they would have to come in the privacy of my room. God and I alone would see them.

Peter was to leave at noon. Robbie, our pastor, came by about 11 AM and asked why I was not going to tell Peter goodbye. I told him I was sure Peter would cry, which would make me cry, and I did not want that to happen. Pastor gave me a long look and said, "I understand," although the look he gave me said, "Who do you think you're fooling?"

I went through the day without shedding a tear. That night I went to bed and finally fell asleep. Three hours later I woke up, realizing I would not see Peter walking through the door again. I would miss the long conversations, the routine phone calls. And then the tears came.

For a week I felt shaky, was unable to function, and had no appetite. I knew something was wrong with me but did not know what it was. I also lost five pounds. Of course I was happy with that. About the seventh day, God spoke to my heart: "You are grieving." God allowed me to grieve, because He knew that Peter would not return in 45 days, not in a year.

Chapter 19

It is important
to let God be the keeper of our hearts. He never fails.

During this period, I called my friend Dottie: "Dottie, I know what's wrong with me. I am going through all the stages of grief!"

"For heaven's sakes, Renee, you are 72 years old; you are not dead. If you did not tell people your age, no one would believe it. They would think you were 62. You are a vibrant, active woman. Peter did not need any help from you in finding a companion. Telling you he needed your help was his excuse to have you in his company outside the church. It would give the two of you a chance to get to know each other. And it did.

"Of course you're grieving! You are in love with Peter. You are in denial. All you have to do is admit it, and you will be all right. Renee, you are not the person today that you were when I met you 15 years ago. The past four months I watched you change from a prude to a very jolly, happy person."

"I am not a prude!"

"You *are* a prude. You are a prude, you are a prude, you are a prude, and I am not taking it back. I had no idea you could be such an open minded, fun person to be with. I get angry with you, Renee; you put everyone before yourself. You are always running around loving, caring for, and waiting on people. God wants you to have some of the love and care you so freely give to others. I watched Peter each Sunday when he walked through the church door. He would look around until his eyes fell on you. All that talk about looking for a companion, but it was you he wanted.

"The two of you were good for each other. But I believe he was hurt because you did not go say goodbye in person, and I am angry with you for not going. How could you not go, Renee?"

"I wanted to go, Dottie. I wanted very much to go. But I just could not bring myself to do it. I did not know what it was to be lonely until Peter left. It is a feeling I have not experienced for many years. I do know that this too shall pass."

❧

The gate to the community was finally up and operating, and I wanted to call Peter's sons to let them know they would need new access cards to get inside the gate. But I didn't have either son's phone number. Since Harold, one of Peter's sons, had signed the church registry when he visited, I called that number and left a message. Two weeks later, I saw Harold at Peter's house and went to apologize for taking that liberty.

"I was not aware that you called," he said. "I have just returned from India, since we did not want Dad to travel alone. We spent a week looking for housing for him. Since we were unable to find suitable housing, he settled in with his sister. He has made contact with a cousin and they are making plans for the winter."

After other conversation he said, "I like the advice you give my dad. Here—let me give you his phone number."

"No, I would not feel comfortable calling someone's home without their permission. But if your dad likes, he may call me."

∾

In December, I wrote Peter a letter and sent it to his home in the village, since I assumed he would return soon. The village's newsletter was also mailed to him, since Peter always wanted to know what went on in the meetings when he was not there. The letter read:

> Hello Peter,
> Numerous people here in the villa and at church have asked about you. I saw Harold on Saturday and spoke with him. I was delighted to learn that you were well settled in and making plans for the winter. It was like a balm, ushering in the love, warmth, and sunshine of God's presence.
>
> We are thankful that God gave you traveling grace and allowed you to arrive safely at your destination. We pray that God's healing angels will place their loving arms around you and keep you in good health so that you may enjoy lots of love and laughter.
>
> The day of your departure was very difficult for me. You are missed.
>
> Our prayers are that God will keep you and yours and permit you to return safely.
>
> Be healthy. Be loved. Be happy!
>
> Renee

∾

In mid-January, I saw Perry's car at his dad's home and went to give him a church bulletin that mentioned his dad. Perry then gave me his contact information, in case I needed to call him. I told Perry that many of the people in the community and at church were asking about his father, and some were disappointed that they had not heard from him, not even a postcard. I said to Perry, "I told them that if they did not hear from your father by the end of New Year's, they probably would not hear from him." When Perry heard that, he looked at me with raised eyebrows but said nothing.

A few weeks later, I saw Perry with a surveyor at his dad's place. The man was measuring off the footage of land. My sister could see them from her window and called me so I could go speak with Perry.

Is your father coming back?" I asked.

"Yes! Oh yes, he will be back in the spring. With the SARS epidemic in the airports, we are afraid to expose him now."

I then explained to Perry that his father had numerous photos of my family, and I would not want Peter to move without returning them to me. Perry asked if I wanted to go inside Peter's house and look for them. I replied, "I do not wish to look through his belongings. It is not that urgent, if he will be returning in a few months. I can wait."

⚘

One day I was surprised when I went to the door to see Perry standing there.

"Hi, Renee," he said, "I've been meaning to stop by to see you but have been very busy working." I invited him in, and he explained, "We have put in a computer for Dad. As soon as the telephone wires are connected, he will be contacting everyone."

I showed Perry my deluxe computer that my son had bought me, even though I was still learning how to use it. Perry replied, "As soon as dad's phone is in, I will come over so we can email him from here." I was shocked; with emphasis I said, "And won't that be a surprise?" With equal emphasis, Perry replied, "Yes, won't it!"

But Perry never came to email his dad from my home, and he never mentioned it the numerous times I saw him. Since it was he who made the suggestion, I did not ask for it.

∾

Another day as I returned from the shopping mall, I found myself stopped at a train crossing. I looked in the rear view mirror and saw a man crouching down as if he did not wish to be seen. I said to myself, "That man looks just like Perry." My Buick had my last name on the license plate; I wondered if he recognized my name and did not wish to be seen. This made me determined to see if it was really Perry. All I had to do was go look in the trunk of my car, which would allow me to see his license plate, which I knew had *his* first name on it.

As soon as I opened my door, the man opened his. Indeed it was Perry! We made small talk as the train came to an end. He said he had spoken to his dad, who was in good health and walking a mile a day. He asked if I would put the pastor's email address in his mailbox for his father; I did as he asked.

∾

One Sunday after dinner, everyone had gone home, except my daughter-in-law Soon-Na and Lucinda and Lisa, my now-grown granddaughters. With all three looking somber, Soon-Na said, "Mama, we want to ask you something. What do you intend to do about Peter?"

"Why would you ask me something like that? What are you talking about?" I countered with a shocked expression.

Lucinda, immediately coming to her mother's rescue, replied, "We told Mama that Peter likes you, and we believe you like him!"

"Is that what you think?"

"That's what we think, Granny!" the girls replied in unison.

I smiled with amusement; it seemed I was transparent to everyone except myself. I responded, "The last time I saw Peter, he said that he wanted me to go with him to London when he returns. What do you think about that?"

I could not believe when they unanimously chimed, "We think you should go!"

"Mama," said Soon-Na, "you worry about everyone's happiness. We think you should start caring about your own. You should be traveling and doing things for yourself—not waiting on everyone else."

It made me feel very good to know that my children and babies cared about my happiness. I could not believe they would be willing to see me leave the country with a man we knew little or nothing about. When Lisa said, "Granny, if that would make you happy, it will make us happy," I felt full inside.

Then I reminded them, "Peter will be returning with a companion."

"No, Granny! We do not believe that," countered Lisa.

"Believe it," I said, "He told me he would."

The girls were quiet for awhile until Lucinda finally asked, "Granny, did he really tell you that?"

"Yes! Yes he did. But Peter admired you girls. I am sure it would please him to know that he met with your approval."

We all laughed. But seven months later, seeing how Peter had never corresponded, they stopped asking about him.

∿

The next time I saw Perry getting his dad's mail, it was mid-July. I told him his father had emailed the pastor three times, but when Pastor tried to return the message, the computer read "faulty email."

Perry raised his eyebrows, saying, "That could not be." He then said he would contact the pastor if I could send him Pastor's phone number. I mailed him Pastor's phone number, but Perry never bothered to call.

∿

One day in August, we held a baby shower for my niece. Six cars had to be parked in Peter's driveway, and Marion and I thought, "If Perry comes today, there will be no place for him to park." He had, however, told me that we should feel free to use the driveway whenever we needed.

Before we could finish our sentence, Perry drove through the gates with a puzzled look on his face. I went over to speak to him and asked about his dad. "He probably will not be coming back until spring," he explained. "We are going there in November. I want to thank you, Renee, for your help."

I told Perry, "I just started a letter to you, but now that I see you, I can tell you its content. There is no need to send it now."

He said, "Send me the letter, anyway." So later I did. Part of it read:

> I want to ask something of you. I made a large collage; it hangs in my hallway. Five generations. Most people are impressed with it, and so was your dad. He asked me for photos of my immediate family, people who attended the church, faces that he knew. He was to make a small collage for me on his computer. He promised to take good care of the photos and return them. Time did not permit your father to get it done.
>
> The photos hold precious memories for me. I would not want to lose them. If your dad decides not to return, I would appreciate it if you would look them up for me.
>
> Also, the church secretary wishes to do a direct mailing from the church to your father in India. She asked if I would ask you for his address. I told her no, I could not do that. It is at her request I send you her name and how she may be reached.

At the shower, Pastor was in the clubhouse, so I went and told him Perry was outside. I knew that he was concerned that he could not respond to Peter's email. It bothered him that he did not know if Peter was told of his attempt to reply.

Perry, in high spirits, said his father was doing well, his skin looked well, and they had pictures from him. He then said, "We believe India is the best place for him; he has lots of relatives and friends there. Of course, it is his call. We will go in November, so who knows—he might return with us. I really appreciate you all. My father was very lonely until he met you."

Pastor explained to Perry that he tried to respond to Peter's email but was unsuccessful. Perry said he did not understand how that could be and asked Pastor to give him his phone number again, so he could call and tell him why his response did not go through. I left the two of them talking and went back inside, thinking that everything Peter had told me was coming to pass. There was a ring of finality in Perry's voice. Pastor never heard from Perry.

❦

A few weeks later, my son Gamal was changing the light bulb over the garage door. As I brought out a new bulb, Perry walked out of his father's house. We met halfway and greeted each other with the usual hug. I said to him, "Come with me. I want to show you something."

Inside my home, I showed him the collage of five family generations. It was important to me for Perry to see it with his own eyes so that he would know that my family photos were in his father's possession.

Perry responded, "I know the photos you are talking about. They are in a manila envelope."

He looked at the collage; it seemed to me his eyes lingered on the largest picture, an old one of me in my nurse's uniform. He said, "These are very nice pictures. I can see the resemblance."

I asked, "So how is your dad?" Perry spoke in a dry, toneless voice: "It has been a while since I spoke to him. He'll be back. He'll be back. The weather is getting cold, so he will not return until spring. Nothing is right; everything is going wrong." He looked drained, sad. I did not ask any questions.

After Perry was gone, Dietra, who had been watching from a distance, asked, "What's bothering Perry?"

"How could I know?" I answered, "I did not question him."

"I just asked because he's usually so bubbly about what a great time his dad is having. You do agree he looked troubled?"

"Yes, I agree."

Chapter 20

About two weeks later, I found a message on my voicemail. I could not believe my ears: a call from Peter's son Harold! I could not comprehend the reason for receiving a call from him, since I had not spoken to or seen him in nearly a year. The message seemed strange, asking for information that he could have easily gotten from his brother Perry:

> Hi, Renee. This is Harold, Peter's son. I hope you are well. I am calling for two reasons: one, I spoke to my dad last week; he has changed homes a couple of times and has not had access to a computer. There had been difficulty with the telephones. Matter of fact, I have not spoken to him for a couple of months. He is finally caught up. I wanted to tell you that.
>
> The second thing is that I would like to get some numbers of the condo associations from you, if you have them. We are at this point probably going to put his condo up for sale. If you get a chance, give me a call at this number. Hope you are doing well.

When Harold and I spoke, I gave him the phone number of the association president. He then said that his father had purchased a home in India and would resume his residency there. I asked him if his father had found the companion he was looking for.

"Yes!" he replied. "He met her at a wedding in April and was introduced to her by a close family member. At first we had some concerns because of her age, but she has some needs and he has some needs, so not much damage can be done."

He said his father would return in the spring to decide what he wanted shipped to India, and he would be bringing his companion. "We are hoping we can get the place sold before he arrives," he explained. "You will get to meet his companion."

When I told Harold about the photos that were in his father's possession, he asked if Perry had been told about them. I said he had. Harold responded, "I don't understand why he has not given them to you. If you want something done, you do not tell Perry. He is working much too hard. Get a pencil. Let me give you my address and phone number. You may call me any time. I would like to have your address, also. It will be nice to keep in touch and send cards during the holidays."

The next morning, I called the association president to let him know that I had given Harold his number.

"Under the circumstance, it was okay," the president said. "What happened? Peter told me he would be gone only 45 days."

"I do not have the answer to that."

Chapter 21

The next day, my daughter Bette called, crying hysterically. She had just received serious results from a diagnostic test.

She sobbed, "I know I should not be mad with God, because He has been so good to me, but I don't think I can bear much more!"

I quietly began to pray, "Oh Jehovah God, you said in your Word in Hebrews 13:5:

I will never leave thee nor forsake thee.

"I need You now, oh Holy Father. I need Your comfort, Your strength. I need to be able to transfer that comfort to my child. I need You. I need You. Speak to my heart, Lord. Give me the words to give to her."

Bette continued, "You cannot possibly understand, Mom. Everything you ever wanted you have had. You have not known great disappointments."

"Sweetheart," I replied, "You do not know the magnitude of the many pains and disappointments I've known. I had to keep a smile on my face. My first concern was always for all of you, my children. Raising you alone was not easy."

"Yes, Mom, we knew there were times when you were hurting, but because you never complained, we pretended we did not know." I could hear her sniffling.

"Two weeks ago, Bette, I shared with you the one thing in life I wanted but never had: to have the man in my life tell me he loved me unconditionally and to act as if he did. I had three husbands. Not one ever acted or stated he loved me unconditionally. They told me they loved me, but it was not enough.

"I did not tell you before, but I tell you now: God granted me that wish through Peter. He gave that to me. Peter was very verbal in stating his feelings for me, but I would always just respond with silence. I would smile and say nothing."

There was silence on the other end of the phone—no sniffling or crying.

I also said, "There was no sex between Peter and me. The friendship we shared was healing. He made me smile inside."

Finally Bette spoke: "It was obvious to all of us that he cared for you, Mama, and I was aware you cared for him."

"You are joking! What did I do wrong? I thought I had my feelings under cover!"

Bette roared with laughter: "Well, you did a poor job! It was in your voice; whenever you spoke of Peter, there was a tenderness I never heard you use for anyone else... So when will he be back?"

"He will not be returning to the village to live," I explained. I then told her about Harold's phone call the day before.

Bette had completely forgotten how hysterical she was when she first called. She had completely forgotten about herself. In retrospect, I thought that my sharing was healing for her. If that were true, my sharing can be healing for others.

I then said to Bette, "I think I will finish the book I started."

"I am so happy to hear you say that, Mom."

❧

That night on the way to Bible class with Robbie, my pastor, I shared with him the events of the past two days. I told him how I shared with Bette, and how I thought it was good for her.

"I am going to finish the book," I told him.

"Do as God lead you," he replied. Then he continued: "Renee, I could not tell you this before now. Soon after Peter came to the church, he asked me to speak to you on his behalf. I told him I could not do that. If it was meant to be, he should just let it happen. Whenever I went to visit him, you were his constant conversation. He was very verbal about how he felt about you. I am sure his children were aware of how he felt. I believe the reason he did not return in 45 days is because they wanted to get him away from you. You are the reason there has been no communication. That is what I believe."

It felt very good to hear this from Robbie, who had never said one word about this until now. However, about three months after Peter and I met, I mentioned to my friend Dottie, "I believe Peter has voiced an interest in me to Pastor."

"Did Pastor tell you that?" she asked.

"No!"

"Did you ask him?"

"No! I would never question Pastor."

"Well, what makes you think that?"

"It's something I feel, Dottie, I feel it in my spirit. I cannot explain it." The Holy Spirit had revealed it to me.

I was disappointed that Peter would not be returning, but I was not surprised. Much of what he told me had come to pass.

❧

Later, as Dottie and I were talking and laughing about our experiences in life, she said, "Renee, wouldn't you just like to wring Peter's neck?"

"Oh, no, no, Dottie," I answered, "I wish him good health and happiness. When you care for your friends, you want them to be happy."

"Only you would say something like that, Renee. Well, you are my friend. I want happiness for you. The two of you were good for each other."

"Dottie, I have good health and am happy."

"But I would have loved to see you go to London."

"It might have been a nice experience, but I have no desire to go to London. I pray every day that God's will be done in my life. If it is in God's plan for me to see London, then in His time, I will go there."

Chapter 22

The last three years that I've lived in the Gardens, I've hosted Sunday dinners at my house, which is five minutes from church. Everyone looks forward to it. Sometimes they say, "Don't you get tired of cooking?" And I tell them, "No. No, I don't." When I moved to the Gardens, I said that I wanted my home to be a haven for others. So I don't turn anyone away, even if it's crowded. I say, "No, come on! Come." It's important to do things for people. I guess they think I have a lot to say.

All the people who had a positive effect on my life helped me to be critical in a loving way. My guests don't see it as being ugly. Usually when I say something, they look at me with amazement, because I hit it right on the mark. They ask, "How did you know that? You were right, but how did you know?" So it makes them want to come back to pick my brain.

The young men who come are all young, good-looking, and single, and I tell them things they don't readily hear from their parents. One of their parents once hugged me and said, "Thank you, thank you! They wouldn't accept that from me."

I remember one Sunday when almost everyone had gone home and only Phillip, Gamal, and I were left. Tall, dark, educated, and familiar with the Word of God, Phillip longed to have a family.

We talked about what a person looks for when selecting a mate. Phillip explained, "When you have a beautiful young lady on your arm, you are making a statement to the world. You can smile and say, 'Look at me. Look at what I have.'"

I replied, "And what do you have? How can we tell what you have just by looking?"

Phillip did not speak but just looked at me. I went on, "When unselfish love finds you, it comes with every component in place. Ask God to give you this kind of love. Be willing to give the same in return. Do not give God instructions on her color, size, length of hair, look, or status. Trust God to make that decision for you.

"I think of the children who long to have a dad in their lives. Think of the joy and happiness you could bring to a little girl. She would call you 'Dad' while you assist her with balancing her bicycle without the training wheels.

"Think of the joy a little boy will get and the pride you will find when he calls you 'Dad' while accompanying you to the golf course.

"God adopted you into His kingdom. You have the power to adopt children into a family. Your living will not have been in vain."

Phillip gave me a long hard stare, then smiled broadly. "I'm impressed. You should dedicate a chapter of your book to counseling and advising. But it's too late for me, Renee."

"God is never late," I replied. "He is always on time—*His* time!"

❧

Of all the things King Solomon, the wisest man of his time, asked of God, He asked for understanding and wisdom.

If you believe that beauty, happiness, or love is found in a pretty or handsome face, you lack wisdom. A beautiful face and flowing hair, a handsome face with the bronze body of a weightlifter, an ugly face with no special features, the average face with average qualities—they are all one and the same. A shell. A covering for what is inside.

Think of a pecan from the supermarket, polished and refined. You crack it open to find it is dried up, dark, and rotten. You are disappointed, because it looked so good on the outside. Then you pick up a pecan from underneath a pecan tree. It is dirty, dusty, and unpolished, but when you crack it open and find rich, succulent meat, your mouth waters.

My grandmother used to quote the saying, "You will find more happiness and benefits being treated like a princess by a toad than you will in being treated like a toad by a Prince."

Some years ago I remember a young man talking to an elderly minister. When she asked him when he was going to get married, he said he could not find the right person. I will never forget her reply: "At the end of the rainbow there is a pot of gold sitting at your feet, and you are missing it, chasing other rainbows."

He gave her a blank look. I don't think he fully understood the depth of what she was saying.

✧

Let me introduce you to Jason, a young man very close to me.

Jason was an only child raised in an upscale suburb who went to good schools and was given the best. He dated Janice, a sweet, soft-spoken young lady who wore glasses and had short hair.

Janice, who lived in an area even more upscale than Jason, adored Jason. But Jason was enraptured with long, flowing hair. He also dated another young lady who had long, flowing hair (as well as a questionable reputation). When Jason's mother asked him why he didn't prefer Janice, he answered, "Her hair does not move when she walks." His mother could not believe that this was his criterion for selecting a girlfriend.

For graduation Jason was given a trip to Hawaii, then enrolled in college when he returned. Feeling that he was a man now, he went full speed ahead, chasing women with long, flowing hair. He began running with the wrong crowd, got himself in serious trouble with the police, and literally ruined his life. As I write these words, Jason is living from shelter to shelter. His life is in shambles, and his parents are heartbroken.

Janice went on to college to pursue a career in medicine and at this writing is doing extremely well.

Sometimes we let our own self-interest overshadow God's plan for our lives; because we do not see their wings, we miss the angel encounters God sends to us. Let go! Let God be in control, replace your will with His will, and you will be wonderfully blessed. Then you will hear him when He says, "You belong to Me. All that you are, all that you have, all that you ever hope to be—you owe it all to Me."

Chapter 23

I sat down at the computer to retrieve my email for the evening, and there was a message from my goddaughter, Allie:

Dear Mama Renee,

I had to write this. I could never say it to you face-to-face, since I couldn't get past the tears of love. Yesterday after dinner when we were all listening to you, I truly saw an angel. As you talked to the boys about unconditional love, I saw an absolutely beautiful woman who literally glowed with beauty. I was stunned into silence.

To myself I said, "She is really beautiful. She's healthy, looks good in all her clothes, still gets around like a 20-year old, and does things for her church, friends, community, and family." I thought, "Peter, you foolish man! You let such a beautiful lady get away. Some day you will regret your decision— if you haven't already."

I ask God why He lets you hurt. I try to say it's because if you had a husband, you would focus on him more, and a lot of us would be lost without your genuine love and care. So God can't let you have a mate. Not yet, anyway. He has to allow you to be able to be shared among so many. I thank God for you, my angel."

Allie

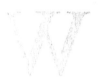

Epilogue

When I told Allie that I was going to write this book, her eyes filled with tears, and she said, "Telling your story will surely be a blessing to many, as it was when you shared just a portion with me. I will remember all my life how you shared with me; you will never know what strength it gave. That through it all, you didn't allow the horrible things others did to you change you.

"You still have nothing but love to give to others. You didn't let bitterness, regret, or revenge steal your life. Knowing how you responded to each crisis encouraged me to continue to do the right things, regardless of what anyone does to me. It inspired me to keep God in my heart first and foremost, and I'll be all right. It also gave me hope that someday, even as I mature, I might find that special someone, because I don't have to just hurt; I can maybe still be loved, too."

❧

Having heard these words spoken to my heart, I write these pages, making myself transparent to the world and believing with all my heart that these words will be a blessing, a balm, and a healing to someone. Long before I was mentally aware of it, God's grace, mercy, and love covered me, and it is my desire to be used by Him.

About the Author

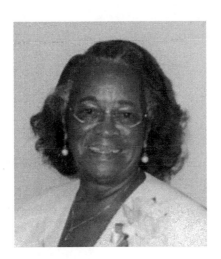

R osella Hayes is a retired Registered Nurse with 28 years experience at the University of Chicago Hospital. She is also a member of the South Suburban Church of God in Homewood, IL, where she is the Chairperson of the Usher Board and the Ordinance Board.

A much-loved mother, grandmother, great-grandmother, godmother, and friend, her love for music is known to all who know her.